MANIPULATION OF THE
SPINE, THORAX AND PELVIS

For Elsevier:

Publisher: Sarena Wolfaard
Development Editor: Fiona Conn
Project Manager: Jagannathan Varadarajan and Anne Dickie
Design: Charles Gray

MANIPULATION OF THE
SPINE, THORAX AND PELVIS

AN OSTEOPATHIC PERSPECTIVE

THIRD EDITION

 With accompanying DVD-ROM

Peter Gibbons MB BS DO DM-SMed MHSc
Adjunct Associate Professor, Department of Rehabilitation Sciences, College of Allied Health,
Oklahoma University Health Science Center, USA

Philip Tehan DO DipPhysio MHSc
Adjunct Associate Professor, School of Biomedical and Health Sciences,
Victoria University, Australia
Adjunct Associate Professor, Department of Rehabilitation Sciences, College of Allied Health,
Oklahoma University Health Science Center, USA

Foreword by

Philip E Greenman DO FAAO
Emeritus Professor, Department of Osteopathic Manipulative Medicine
and Emeritus Professor of Physical Medicine & Rehabilitation,
Michigan State University College of Osteopathic Medicine

Photographs by
Tim Turner

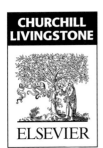

CHURCHILL
LIVINGSTONE

ELSEVIER

Edinburgh London New York Oxford Philadelphia St Louis Sydney Toronto 2010

CHURCHILL
LIVINGSTONE
ELSEVIER

First Edition © Harcourt Publishers Limited 2000
Second Edition © Elsevier Science Limited 2006
Third Edition © Elsevier Limited 2010

ISBN 978 0 7020 3130 4
  Reprinted 2010 (twice)

British Library Cataloguing in Publication Data
A catalogue record for this book is available from the British Library

Library of Congress Cataloging in Publication Data
A catalog record for this book is available from the Library of Congress

Notice
Neither the Publisher nor the Authors assume any responsibility for any loss or injury and/or damage to persons or property arising out of or related to any use of the material contained in this book. It is the responsibility of the treating practitioner, relying on independent expertise and knowledge of the patient, to determine the best treatment and method of application for the patient.

The Publisher

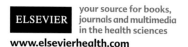
Printed in China

Contents

The DVD-ROM accompanying this text includes video sequences of all the techniques described in Part B (with the exception of the last technique described in Chapter 11). These are indicated in the text by the following symbol. To look at the video for a given technique, click on the relevant icon in the contents list on the DVD-ROM.

The DVD-ROM is designed to be used in conjunction with the text and not as a stand-alone product.

Contents

Foreword

HVLA (High Velocity Low Amplitude) thrust technique is one of the oldest and most commonly used manipulative techniques, practiced by a variety of health care practitioners.

The third edition of this text brings much new information on the technique to the reader. Currently there is consensus on the need for more evidence in order to practice evidence-based medicine (EBM). The authors have done an exemplary job in providing current evidence for the HVLA thrust technique in new and updated references throughout the text.

The book is divided into three parts, and it is in Part A that the majority of the new supporting evidence is found, with 130 new references in total. For example, Chapter 3 provides an excellent analysis of the controversial field of coupled motion of the spine bringing in the newest research information and in chapter 5 current knowledge in the area of safety and HVLA thrust techniques is greatly expanded, with over fifty new citations added. Forty new citations support the rationale for the use of HVLA thrust techniques in Chapter 6.

Part B covers the HVLA thrust techniques themselves in a fashion that can serve both the novice and the expert. They are well illustrated and easily understood: what remains for the reader is practice. Hand skills in manipulation are like the skill in playing a musical instrument such as the piano. It takes many hours, even years, to acquire the ability to play Chopin and this applies to manipulation skills as well. The accompanying DVD is most helpful in demonstrating the techniques discussed in Part B.

Part C offers the reader a quick but comprehensive understanding of treatment failures. When applied appropriately to the right diagnosis on the right patient, these techniques should be painless, safe and effective.

HVLA thrust techniques have been found to be effective in a large variety of musculoskeletal conditions. For your patient they may well be an answer to pain and suffering. Read, study, practice and enjoy this significant contribution to the field of manipulative therapies: your patient will appreciate it.

Philip E. Greenman, DO, FAAO
Emeritus Professor
Osteopathic Manipulative Medicine
Emeritus Professor
Physical Medicine & Rehabilitation
Michigan State University

Preface

This third edition of *Manipulation of the Spine, Thorax and Pelvis: An Osteopathic Perspective* has been produced at a time of increasing knowledge related to the use of manipulative techniques in clinical practice, and has been updated accordingly. The move towards an evidence-based and patient-centred approach to healthcare requires the modern practitioner to utilize the best available evidence to inform clinical practice, to be cognizant of the legal and ethical requirements for informed consent and to use the appropriate instruments to monitor patient progress, and the third edition reflects these requirements of practice.

Patient comfort and safety remain major considerations when selecting a treatment approach. Thrust techniques have been considered potentially more dangerous compared with other osteopathic techniques, particularly those relating to the cervical spine, but current evidence indicates that the risks of manipulation for spinal pain are very low, provided patients are assessed and selected for treatment by trained practitioners.

Cervical artery dissection should always be considered in the differential diagnosis of patients presenting with headache and / or neck pain. The text has been updated to embrace current research findings and recommendations regarding pre-treatment risk assessment relating to both the vertebral and internal carotid arteries. Most of the research and reporting of both transient and more serious complications of manual interventions have focused upon high-velocity low-amplitude (HVLA) thrust techniques so we have expanded the text to review relative risks of thrust and non-thrust techniques. The evidence base for the use of spinal manipulation in patients with disc lesions has been updated, as the application of thrust techniques in these patients remains controversial.

Our goal remains to present a text that will provide the necessary information relating to all aspects of the delivery of HVLA thrust techniques in one comprehensive volume, so that practitioners can use these techniques safely and in the appropriate circumstances. Since the second edition, additional research and guidelines have been published that support the use of HVLA thrust techniques, and these have been incorporated into the third edition. Psychological and social influences on spinal pain and disability have also been explored in more depth.

For a commonly used treatment approach, it is surprising that there are such limited resources to support learning and skill refinement in HVLA thrust techniques. Most of the learning of HVLA thrust techniques has been dependent upon personal instruction and demonstration. There are still only a handful of osteopathic technique books and manuals and few of these relate solely to thrust techniques.

The material presented in this text was developed in response to the learning needs of undergraduate and postgraduate students over a 35-year period. The novice has to acquire basic skills and experienced practitioners should reflect upon their performance and constantly refine each thrust technique. It has been our experience that the structured step-by-step format used in the text and the visual reinforcement offered by the accompanying

DVD-ROM have been successful in assisting both initial development and subsequent refinement of the psychomotor skills necessary for the effective delivery of HVLA thrust techniques. Experience has shown that the video images included on the DVD-ROM have proved useful for both students and practitioners. The third edition DVD-ROM has been updated and expanded to clarify the principles of spinal positioning and locking using a coupled motion model.

Peter Gibbons, Philip Tehan
Melbourne 2010

Acknowledgements

As in the first and second editions, we are grateful to those colleagues who knowingly or unknowingly assisted in the development of the book. We also acknowledge that the constant questioning by undergraduate and postgraduate students has contributed significantly to the development of the material in the text.

Tim Turner has provided the photographs for all editions. We would like to thank him for his patience and understanding during the many photographic sessions. We are again indebted to Andrea Robertson for her good humour and endurance during the long sessions spent as the model for the photographs and DVD-ROM. We greatly appreciate the assistance of Dr Frank Burke (Consultant Radiologist) in providing access to imaging facilities and advice regarding the fluoroscopic images of the lumbar spine and to Dr John Kwon for providing fluoroscopic images of the cervical spine that appear on the DVD-ROM. The teaching potential of the text has been greatly enhanced by the visual material and their contribution.

A special thanks is extended to Sarena Wolfaard and Fiona Conn at Elsevier for their help, support and encouragement for the third edition.

Most importantly, our greatest debt of gratitude goes to Jill Tehan and Christine Leek whose tireless support made the writing and updating of this book possible.

HVLA thrust techniques – an osteopathic perspective

1

Introduction

Manipulative techniques for the spine, thorax and pelvis are commonly utilized for the treatment of pain and dysfunction. Proficiency in their use requires training, practice and development of palpatory and psychomotor skills. The purpose of this book is to provide a resource that will aid development of the knowledge and skills necessary to perform high-velocity low-amplitude (HVLA) thrust techniques in practice. It is written not just for the novice manipulator but also for any practitioner who uses thrust techniques. While the book presents an osteopathic perspective, it does not promote or endorse any particular treatment model or approach.

The term 'manipulation' is often used to describe a range of manual therapy techniques. This text focuses specifically upon HVLA procedures where the practitioner applies a rapid thrust or impulse. The aim of HVLA thrust techniques is to achieve joint cavitation that is accompanied by a 'popping' or 'cracking' sound. This audible release distinguishes HVLA thrust techniques from other osteopathic manipulative techniques. HVLA thrust techniques are also known by a number of different names, e.g. adjustment, high-velocity thrust, mobilization with impulse and grade V mobilization.

The book is divided into three parts. Part A comprises seven chapters that provide an osteopathic perspective on the use of HVLA thrust techniques and reviews indications, research evidence, kinematics, safety and research.

An overview of the osteopathic philosophy and practice that underpins osteopathic manipulative technique and treatment is presented in Chapter 2. Chapter 3 reviews spinal kinematics and coupled motion of the spine. Practitioners require knowledge of biomechanics and coupled motion characteristics in order to apply the principles of spinal locking used in HVLA thrust techniques. The osteopathic profession has developed a classification of spinal motion. Chapter 4 describes Type 1 and Type 2 movements and the relevance of coupled motion to spinal positioning and joint locking.

Complications of, and contraindications to, HVLA thrust techniques are outlined in Chapter 5. Relative risks of thrust and non-thrust techniques and the use of HVLA thrust techniques in patients with disc lesions are discussed. Pre-manipulative assessment for cervical artery compromise and upper cervical instability is described and the use of testing protocols is reviewed in light of the published literature.

Chapter 6 reviews the literature relating to cavitation, the evidence related to the efficacy of spinal manipulation and outlines a decision-making process that will assist practitioners to determine when a HVLA thrust technique might be used in clinical practice.

Research is necessary to validate the use of osteopathic techniques in clinical practice, including HVLA thrust techniques. Chapter 7 discusses where research should be focused and identifies strategies that can be used by practitioners to classify patients and document patient outcomes.

Part B outlines in detail specific HVLA thrust techniques for the spine, rib cage and pelvis. This part combines photographs and descriptive text that is supported by the video images of HVLA thrust techniques on the accompanying DVD-ROM.

HVLA thrust techniques can be described in terms of bone movement or joint gliding. In this text, all 41 techniques are outlined utilizing the principle of joint gliding. This approach has been shown to be effective in the teaching of HVLA thrust techniques to both undergraduate and postgraduate students.

The text has been designed to provide a logical step-by-step format that has consistency throughout the book. Each technique is described from the moment the patient is positioned on the couch, through a series of steps up to and including segmental localization and delivery of the thrust. Each individual technique is logically organized under a number of specific headings:

- Contact point(s)
- Applicator(s)
- Patient positioning
- Operator stance
- Positioning for thrust
- Adjustments to achieve appropriate pre-thrust tension
- Immediately pre-thrust
- Delivering the thrust.

Individuals use a variety of methods to acquire complex psychomotor skills, with structured and repeated practice a key element in the development and maintenance of proficiency. Experiencing these both as an operator and as a model can enhance the learning of HVLA thrust techniques.

The art of manipulation is very individual, requiring HVLA thrust techniques to be adapted to the needs of both practitioner and patient. While some modification to the described techniques will occur with developing proficiency, the underlying principles remain the same. These principles can be summarized as follows:

1. Exclude contraindications.
2. Obtain informed consent.
3. Ensure patient comfort.
4. Ensure operator comfort and optimum posture.
5. Use spinal locking.
6. Identify appropriate pre-thrust tissue tension.
7. Apply HVLA thrust.

If these principles are applied, HVLA thrust techniques provide a safe and effective treatment option.

A common experience in the evolution of proficiency in thrust techniques is a sense of frustration and impatience when skill development is slow or variable. Experienced practitioners can similarly experience difficulties achieving cavitation in certain circumstances. Part C provides a troubleshooting and self-evaluation guide to identify those problems that may limit the effective application of HVLA thrust techniques.

Integral to the practice of osteopathic medicine is an understanding of the interrelationship of mind, body and environment. Osteopathic treatment encompasses more than joint manipulation alone and this manual represents only part of the art and science of osteopathic medicine.

2

Osteopathic philosophy, practice and technique

Osteopathy, or osteopathic medicine, is a philosophy, a science and an art. Its philosophy embraces the concept of the unity of body structure and function in health and disease. Its science includes the chemical, physical and biological sciences related to the maintenance of health and the prevention, cure and alleviation of disease. Its art is the application of the philosophy and the science in the practice of osteopathic medicine and surgery in all its branches and specialties.

Health is based on the natural capacity of the human organism to resist and combat noxious influences in the environment and to compensate for their effects; to meet, with adequate reserve, the usual stresses of daily life and the occasional severe stresses imposed by extremes of environment and activity.

Disease begins when this natural capacity is reduced, or when it is exceeded or overcome by noxious influences.

Osteopathic medicine recognizes that many factors impair this capacity and the natural tendency towards recovery and that among the most important of these factors are the local disturbances or lesions of the musculoskeletal system. Osteopathic medicine is therefore concerned with liberating and developing all the resources that constitute the capacity for resistance and recovery, thus recognizing the validity of the ancient observation that the physician deals with a patient as well as a disease.[1]

The philosophy underpinning the osteopathic approach to patient care can be enunciated as shown in Box 2.1.

OSTEOPATHIC TREATMENT MODELS

Scientific validation for the use of manual and manipulative approaches, including high-velocity low-amplitude (HVLA) thrust techniques, is limited. Consequently, practitioners must rely upon theoretical and clinical models to justify the use of HVLA thrust techniques in clinical practice.

Osteopaths use five treatment and clinical-reasoning models:[2]

1. Biomechanical
2. Neurological
   a. autonomic nervous system
   b. pain
   c. neuroendocrine
3. Respiratory / circulatory
4. Bioenergy
5. Psychobehavioural.

Box 2.1 Philosophy underpinning osteopathic approach

- The body is an integrated unit
- The body is self-regulating with inherent capacity for healing
- Structure and function are inter-dependent
- Somatic component to disease
- Neuromusculoskeletal dysfunction impacts on overall health status
- Neuromusculoskeletal dysfunction impacts on recovery from injury and disease
- Unhindered fluid interchange necessary for maintenance of health

---

Biomechanical (postural / structural)

This model is based upon the concept that mechanical and structural dysfunction can result from single incidences of trauma or from microtrauma occurring over time and as a result of postural imbalance or occupational and environmental stresses. Cumulative microtrauma can lead to a breakdown of the body's normal compensatory mechanisms with resultant development of dysfunction and pain.

The biomechanical model requires the practitioner to restore maximum function to the neuromusculoskeletal system with enhancement of the body's ability to compensate for external mechanical stresses and any primary or secondary postural imbalance. Therapy is directed towards restoring near-normal motion and / or function to joints, ligaments, muscles and fascia. The aim is to regain optimal function within the musculoskeletal system.

Neurological

This model is based upon the concept that neural mechanisms may be influenced by the use of manual medicine approaches. The neurological models provide a framework for treatment that is based upon postulated mechanisms of interaction between the somatic and neurological systems. These mechanisms are complex and beyond the scope of this manual. It is suggested that manual intervention may influence:

- the two divisions of the autonomic nervous system
- the integration of function between the central and peripheral nervous systems for modulation of pain
- the neuroendocrine–immune connection, resulting in both local and systemic effects.

Respiratory / circulatory

This model is based upon the concept that normal fluid exchange is essential for the continued health of tissues at both the 'micro' and 'macro' level. Manual treatment is directed towards improving blood and lymph flow and aiding intracellular fluid exchange by enhancing musculoskeletal function. Treatment is directed towards restoring the capacity of the musculoskeletal system to assist venous and lymphatic return.

Bioenergy

This model is based upon the body's inherent energy fields that can be utilized for diagnosis and treatment. Internal and external environmental factors may influence the vitality and quality of energy flow within the human body. The aim of treatment is to restore balance and harmony to these fields of energy.

Psychobehavioural

This model recognizes that many internal and external factors influence a patient's response to pain and dysfunction. Social, economic and cultural factors all impact upon the way in which a patient deals with pain, dysfunction and disability. An understanding of the factors that can influence a patient's coping mechanisms is pivotal to this model, as is knowledge of the psychosocial interventions that may assist the patient to deal with pain and disability.

These five models provide a conceptual framework upon which decisions relating to patient management can be made. It must be understood that these are simply conceptual models with various amounts of evidence to support their use.

These osteopathic models provide a framework for choosing a treatment approach and selecting osteopathic manipulative techniques. However, the treatment models do not clearly establish a rationale for the use of HVLA thrust techniques as distinct from other osteopathic manipulative techniques.

DIAGNOSIS OF SOMATIC DYSFUNCTION

Osteopaths diagnose somatic dysfunction by searching for abnormal function within the somatic system.

Palpation is fundamental to structural and functional diagnosis.[3]

The accepted definition for somatic dysfunction in the 'Glossary of osteopathic terminology' is as follows:

Somatic dysfunction is an impaired or altered function of related components of the somatic (body framework) system: skeletal, arthrodial and myofascial structures, and related vascular, lymphatic, and neural elements.[4]

Research has explored both inter- and intra-examiner reliability of various diagnostic palpatory procedures. Inter-examiner reliability consists of one assessment of all subjects by each of two or more raters, blinded to each other's observations, and allows assessment of rater agreement. Intra-examiner reliability is determined by repeated measurements of single individuals to evaluate rater self-consistency.

Osteopaths have shown reasonable levels of inter-examiner agreement for passive gross motion testing on selected subjects with consistent findings of regional motion asymmetry.[5,6] One osteopathic study demonstrated low agreement of findings for patients with acute spinal complaints when practitioners used their own diagnostic procedures.[7] Level of agreement can be improved by negotiating and selecting specific tests for detecting patient improvement.[8] Standardization of testing procedures can improve both inter- and intra-examiner reliability.[9]

In asymptomatic somatic dysfunction, high levels of inter- and intra-observer agreement for palpatory findings have yet to be demonstrated. Many studies and systematic reviews indicate that inter- and intra-examiner reliability for palpatory motion testing without pain provocation is poor.[10–21]

Poor reliability of clinical tests involving palpation may be partially explained by error in location of bony landmarks[22] and differences in palpation technique.[23] Consensus training has been demonstrated to improve inter-observer reliability in the palpatory tests of lumbar spine tissue texture and tenderness.[24] Palpation as a diagnostic tool has been reported to demonstrate high levels of sensitivity and specificity in detecting symptomatic intervertebral segments.[25,26] A further study refuted some of these findings demonstrating that manual examination had high sensitivity but poor specificity for identifying cervical zygapophysial joint pain.[27]

A systematic review of manual examination of the spine identified that reproducibility of palpation for pain response was consistently better than for motion palpation.[28] Increasing evidence is emerging that clusters of provocation and motion palpation tests have better reliability than single tests for assessing the sacroiliac joints.[21,29,30]

Traditionally, diagnosis of somatic dysfunction was made on the basis of a number of positive findings. Specific criteria in identifying areas of dysfunction were developed and related to the observational and palpatory findings of asymmetry, altered range of motion, tissue texture changes and tenderness. This was represented as the acronym TART (tissue tenderness, asymmetry, range of motion and tissue texture changes).[2,4,31]

Pain provocation and reproduction of familiar symptoms should also be used to localize somatic dysfunction. The presence of somatic dysfunction and / or pathology should be determined not only by physical examination but also by information gained from a thorough patient history and patient feedback during assessment. This depth of diagnostic deliberation is essential if one is to select which case may or may not be amenable to treatment and which treatment approach might be the most effective while offering the patient a reasoned prognosis. We would advocate that the convention for the diagnosis of somatic dysfunction – TART – should be expanded to include patient feedback relating to pain provocation and the reproduction of familiar symptoms.

Somatic dysfunction is identified by the S-T-A-R-T of diagnosis (Box 2.2)

S   relates to symptom reproduction

Although somatic dysfunction can be asymptomatic, it commonly exists within the context of a patient presenting with symptoms. Pain provocation and the reporting of reproduction of familiar symptoms are therefore essential components of the physical examination.

T   relates to tissue tenderness

Undue tissue tenderness is often present and must be differentiated from reproduction of the patient's familiar pain.

A   relates to asymmetry

DiGiovanna links the criteria of asymmetry to a positional focus stating that the 'position of the vertebra or other bone is asymmetrical'.[31] Greenman broadens the concept of asymmetry by including functional in addition to structural asymmetry.[2]

R   relates to range of motion

Alteration in range of motion can apply to a single joint, several joints or a region of the musculoskeletal system. The abnormality may be either restricted or increased mobility and includes assessment of quality of movement and 'end feel'.

T   relates to tissue texture changes

The identification of tissue texture changes is important in the diagnosis of somatic dysfunction. Palpable changes may be noted in superficial, intermediate and deep tissues. It is important for clinicians to recognize normal from abnormal.

Box 2.2 Diagnosis of somatic dysfunction

- S   relates to symptom reproduction
- T   relates to tissue tenderness
- A   relates to asymmetry
- R   relates to range of motion
- T   relates to tissue texture changes

The diagnosis of somatic dysfunction should not be based upon a single finding but should be determined by the clinician identifying a number of positive findings that are consistent with the patient's clinical presentation (Box 2.3).

Box 2.3 Diagnosis of somatic dysfunction

- Not be based upon a single finding
- Determined by identifying a number of positive findings consistent with the patient's clinical presentation

---

For example, a patient with cervicogenic headaches with related somatic dysfunction might present with restricted active and passive range of movement in the cervical spine; segmental assessment may identify localized movement restriction; palpation may identify muscular hypertonicity and / or undue local tenderness; and examination may reproduce the patient's familiar symptoms.

SOMATIC DYSFUNCTION AND OSTEOPATHIC MANIPULATIVE TECHNIQUES

A patient's overall management requires the identification of broad therapeutic objectives. Models and guidelines for the diagnosis and treatment of low back pain have been developed.[32,33] These approaches have a broad utility and can be generalized to the management of spinal pain. Box 2.4 is a list of objectives in the diagnosis and treatment of spinal disorders.

Patients should be made aware of the potential debilitation of excessive bed rest, the dangers of overmedication and the inadvisability of surgery without strong preoperative indications.

Once a practitioner has established therapeutic objectives, consideration must be given to the specific treatment of somatic dysfunction. Many factors will influence the final composition of the manipulative prescription, as is the case when a physician

Box 2.4 Objectives in the diagnosis and treatment of spinal disorders

- Focused history and clinical examination to classify patients into one of the following categories:
  — mechanical pain with no neurological involvement
  — mechanical pain associated with neurological involvement
  — spinal pain due to serious pathology (red flags)
- Assessment of psychosocial risk factors and barriers to return to normal activity
- Provide information to reassure patients about their condition
- Provide patients with information on effective self-care options
- Provide patients with advice to remain active
- Give priority to treatments of known efficacy

Box 2.5 Osteopathic manipulative techniques

- Articulatory
- Balanced ligamentous tension
- Chapman's reflexes
- Facilitated positional release
- Fascial ligamentous release
- Functional
- HVLA thrust
- Integrated neuromuscular release and myofascial release
- Lymphatic
- Muscle energy
- Myofascial trigger point
- Osteopathy in the cranial field
- Progressive inhibition of neuromuscular structures
- Soft tissue
- Strain and counterstrain
- Visceral

considers a patient's age, weight, drug and allergy history, etc. when prescribing medication. The osteopath similarly takes account of factors such as the patient's age, the acuteness or chronicity of the presenting complaint, general health, response to previous treatment and the osteopath's own training and expertise in the delivery of specific treatment approaches. This list is not exhaustive and many other factors can influence the final selection of manipulative techniques and the frequency of treatment.

When formulating the manipulative prescription, the osteopath has a wide range of techniques to draw upon (Box 2.5).

Some osteopathic techniques are named according to the activating forces used (e.g. muscle energy, springing, or HVLA thrust), whereas other techniques (e.g. strain / counterstrain, myofascial release and osteopathy in the cranial field) refer to a concept of treatment. Techniques are also classified as either direct or indirect techniques. Direct techniques involve the application of force to engage the restrictive barrier, whereas indirect techniques utilize identification of 'freedom' or 'ease' of movement by moving away from the restrictive barrier. Ideally, osteopaths should embrace a range of different techniques and not favour any one specific approach.

In practice, the most commonly used osteopathic manipulative treatment techniques are articulatory, HVLA thrust, counterstrain, muscle energy, myofascial / neuromuscular release and soft tissue techniques.[34] A study of members of the Australian Osteopathic Association identified that high-velocity manipulation was one of the most commonly used forms of osteopathic manipulative treatment.[35]

References

1 Special Committee on Osteopathic Principles and Osteopathic Technic, Kirksville College of Osteopathy and Surgery. An interpretation of the osteopathic concept. Tentative formulation of a teaching guide for faculty, hospital staff and student body. J Osteopathy 1953; 60:8–10.

2 Greenman PE. Principles of Manual Medicine, 3rd edn. Philadelphia, PA: Lippincott Williams & Wilkins; 2003.

3 Kappler RE. Palpatory skills and exercises for developing the sense of touch. In: Ward R ed. Foundations for Osteopathic Medicine, 2nd Edition. Philadelphia: Lippincott Williams & Wilkins; 2003: Ch. 38.

4 The Glossary Review Committee of the Educational Council on Osteopathic Principles. Glossary of osteopathic terminology. In: Allen TW, ed. AOA Yearbook and Directory of Osteopathic Physicians. Chicago: American Osteopathic Association; 1993:Glossary.

5 Johnston WL, Elkiss ML, Marino RV, Blum GA. Passive gross motion testing: Part II. A study of interexaminer agreement. J Am Osteopath Assoc 1982;81(5):65–69.

6 Johnston WL, Beal MC, Blum GA, et al. Passive gross motion testing: Part III. Examiner agreement on selected subjects. J Am Osteopath Assoc 1982;81(5):70–74.

7 McConnell DG, Beal MC, Dinnar U, et al. Low agreement of findings in neuromusculoskeletal examinations by a group of osteopathic physicians using their own procedures. J Am Osteopath Assoc 1980;79(7):59–68.

8 Beal MC, Goodridge JP, Johnston WL, et al. Interexaminer agreement on patient improvement after negotiated selection of tests. J Am Osteopath Assoc 1980;79(7):45–53.

9 Marcotte J, Normand M, Black P. The kinematics of motion palpation and its effect on the reliability for cervical spine rotation. J Manipulative Physiol Ther 2002;25(7):471.

10 Van Duersen LLJM, Patijn J, Ockhuysen AL, et al. The value of some clinical tests of the sacroiliac joint. Man Med 1990;5:96–99.

11 Laslett M, Williams M. The reliability of selected pain provocation tests for sacroiliac joint pathology. In: Leeming A, Mooney V, Dorman T, et al. eds. The Integrated Function of the Lumbar Spine and Sacroiliac Joint. Rotterdam: ECO; 1995:485–498.

12 Gonnella C, Paris S, Kutner M. Reliability in evaluating passive intervertebral motion. Phys Ther 1982;62:436–444.

13 Matyas T, Bach T. The reliability of selected techniques in clinical arthrokinematics. Aust J Physiother 1985;31(5):175–195.

14 Harvey D, Byfield D. Preliminary studies with a mechanical model for the evaluation of spinal motion palpation. Clin Biomechanics 1991;6:79–82.

15 Lewit K, Liebenson C. Palpation – problems and implications. J Manipulative Physiol Ther 1993;16(9):586–590.

16 Panzer DM. The reliability of lumbar motion palpation. J Manipulative Physiol Ther 1992;15(8):518–524.

17 Love RM, Brodeur R. Inter- and intra-examiner reliability of motion palpation for the thoracolumbar spine. J Manipulative Physiol Ther 1987;10(1):1–4.

18 Smedmark V, Wallin M, Arvidsson I. Inter-examiner reliability in assessing passive intervertebral motion of the cervical spine. Man Ther 2000;5(2):97–101.

19 Hestboek L, Leboeuf-Yde C. Are chiropractic tests for the lumbo-pelvic spine reliable and valid? A systematic critical literature review. J Manipulative Physiol Ther 2000;23(4):258–275.

20 Van Trijffel E, Anderegg Q, Bossuyt P, Lucas C. Inter-examiner reliability of passive assessment of intervertebral motion in the cervical and lumbar spine: A systematic review. Man Ther 2005;10(4):256–269.

21 Robinson H, Brox J, Robinson R, et al. The reliability of selected motion and pain provocation tests for the sacroiliac joint. Man Ther 2007;12(1):72–79.

22 O'Haire C, Gibbons P. Inter-examiner and intra-examiner agreement for assessing sacroiliac anatomical landmarks using palpation and observation: A pilot study. Man Ther 2000;5(1):13–20.

23 Holmgren U, Waling K. Inter-examiner reliability of four static palpation tests used for assessing pelvic dysfunction. Man Ther 2008;13(1):50–56.

24 Degenhardt B, Snider K, Snider E, et al. Interobserver reliability of osteopathic palpatory diagnostic tests of the lumbar spine: Improvements from consensus training. J Am Osteopath Assoc 2005;105(10):465–473.

25 Jull G, Bogduk N, Marsland A. The accuracy of manual diagnosis for cervical zygapophysial joint pain syndromes. Med J Aust 1988;148:233–236.

26 Jull G, Zito G, Trott P, et al. Inter-examiner reliability to detect painful upper cervical joint dysfunction. Aust Physiother 1997;43(2):125–129.

27 King W, Lau P, Lees R, et al. The validity of manual examination in assessing patients with neck pain. Spine J 2007;7(1):22–26.

28 Stochkendahl M, Christensen H, Hartvigsen J, et al. Manual examination of the spine: A systematic critical literature review of reproducibility. J Manipulative Physiol Ther 2006;29(6):475–485.

29 Cibulka M, Koldenhoff R. Clinical usefulness of a cluster of sacroiliac joint tests in patients with and without low back pain. J Orthop Sports Phys Ther 1999;29(2):83–89.

30 Arab A, Abdollahi I, Joghataei M, et al. Inter- and intra- examiner reliability of single and composites of selected motion palpation and pain provocation tests for sacroiliac joint. Man Ther 2009 Apr;14(2):213–221.

31 DiGiovanna EL, Schiowitz S. An Osteopathic Approach to Diagnosis and Treatment, 3rd edn. Philadelphia: Lippincott Williams & Wilkins; 2004.

32 Chou R, Qaseem A, Snow V, et al. Diagnosis and treatment of back pain: A joint clinical practice guideline from the American College of Physicians and the American pain Society. Ann Intern Med 2007;147(7):478–491.

33 Poitras S, Rossignol M, Dionne C, et al. An interdisciplinary clinical practice model for the management of low back pain in primary care: The CLIP project. BMC Musculoskeletal Disorders 2008; April 21;9:54.

34 Johnson S, Kurtz M. Osteopathic manipulative treatment techniques preferred by contemporary osteopathic physicians. J Am Osteopath Assoc 2003;103(5):219–224.

35 Orrock P. Profile of members of the Australian Osteopathic Association: Part 1 – The practitioners. Int J Osteopath Med March 2009;12(1):14–24.

3

Kinematics and coupled motion of the spine

Clinicians use palpatory assessment of individual intervertebral segments prior to the application of a thrust technique. The osteopathic profession has used Fryette's model of the physiological movements of the spine to assist in the diagnosis of somatic dysfunction and the application of treatment techniques. Fryette[1] outlined his research into the physiological movements of the vertebral column in 1918. He presented a model that indicated coupled motion occurred in the spine and displayed different coupling characteristics dependent upon spinal segmental level and posture. The muscle energy approach is one system of segmental spinal lesion diagnosis and treatment predicated upon Fryette's Laws.[2] Practitioners utilizing muscle energy technique (MET) use these laws of coupled motion as a predictive model both to formulate a mechanical diagnosis and to select the precisely controlled position required in the application of both muscle energy and thrust techniques. Current literature challenges the validity of Fryette's Laws.

BIOMECHANICS

Convention dictates that intervertebral motion is described in relation to motion of the superior vertebra upon the inferior vertebra. Motion is further defined in relation to the anterior surface of the vertebral body; an example of which would be the direction of vertebral rotation, which is described in relation to the direction in which the anterior surface of the vertebra moves rather than the posterior elements.

In the clinical setting, vertebral motion is described using standard anatomical cardinal planes and axes of the body. Spinal motion can be described as rotation around, and translation along, an axis as the vertebral body moves along one of the cardinal planes. By convention the vertical axis is labelled the y-axis; the horizontal axis is labelled the x-axis; and the antero-posterior axis is the z-axis (Fig. 3.1).[3]

In biomechanical terms, flexion is anterior (sagittal) rotation of the superior vertebra around the x-axis, while there is accompanying forward (sagittal) translation of the vertebral body along the z-axis. In extension, the opposite occurs and the superior vertebra rotates posteriorly around the x-axis and translates posteriorly along the z-axis. In sidebending, there is bone rotation around the antero-posterior z-axis, but sidebending is rarely a pure movement and is generally accompanied by vertebral rotation. The combination, and association, of one movement with others is termed 'coupled motion'. The concept of coupled motion is not recent. As early as 1905, Lovett[4] published his observations of coupled motion of the spine.

COUPLED MOTION

Coupled motion is described by White and Panjabi[5] as a 'phenomenon of consistent association of one motion (translation or rotation) about an axis with another motion about a second axis'. Bogduk and Twomey[3] describe coupled movements as 'movements

13

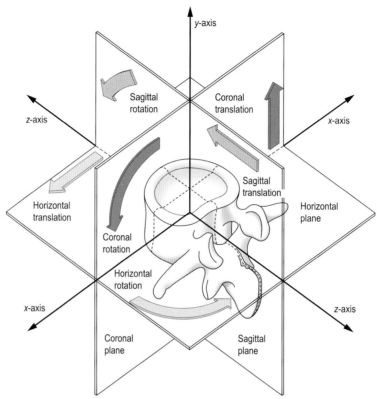

Figure 3.1 Axes of motion.
(Reproduced with permission from Bogduk.[3])

that occur in an unintended or unexpected direction during the execution of a desired motion'. Stokes et al[6] simply state coupling to be when 'a primary (or intentional) movement results in a joint also moving in other directions'. Where rotation occurs in a consistent manner as an accompaniment to sidebending it has been termed conjunct rotation.[7,8] Therefore, in rotation the vertebra should rotate around the vertical y-axis but translation will be complex dependent upon the extent and direction of coupling movements. Coupling will cause shifting axes of motion.

Greenman[9] maintains that rotation of the spinal column is always coupled with sidebending with the exception of the atlanto-axial joint. The coupled rotation can be in the same direction as sidebending (e.g. sidebending right, rotation right) or in opposite directions (e.g. sidebending right, rotation left). The osteopathic profession developed the convention of naming the coupled movements as Type 1 and Type 2 movements (Figs. 3.2 and 3.3).[10]

These concepts of vertebral motion are attributed to Fryette. Fryette acknowledges the contribution made to his understanding of spinal movement by Lovett. Lovett had undertaken research on cadavers in order to understand the structure and aetiology of scoliotic curves.

Fryette acknowledged that Lovett's findings for the thoracic and lumbar spine were correct in the position Lovett had placed the spine for his cadaveric experiments, but maintained they would not be true if the lumbar and thoracic spine were placed in different positions of flexion or extension. Fryette performed his own experiments upon a 'spine mounted in soft rubber' and introduced the concept of neutral (facets not engaged) and non-neutral (facets engaged and controlling vertebral

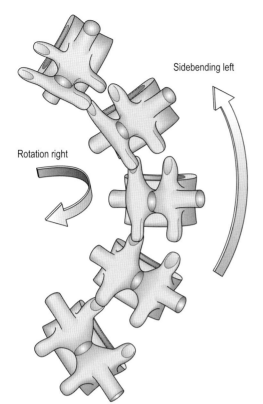

Figure 3.2 Type 1 movement. Sidebending and rotation occur to opposite sides.
(Reproduced with permission from Gibbons and Tehan.[10])

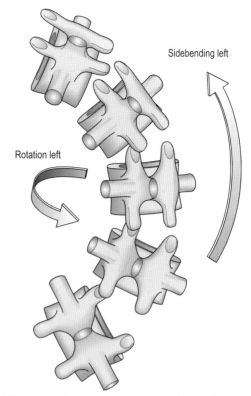

Figure 3.3 Type 2 movement. Sidebending and rotation occur to the same side.
(Reproduced with permission from Gibbons and Tehan.[10])

motion) positioning. Fryette defined neutral 'to mean the position of any area of the spine in which the facets are idling, in the position between the beginning of flexion and the beginning of extension'. In the cervical spine below C2, the facets are considered always to be in a non-neutral position and are therefore assumed to control vertebral motion. The thoracic and lumbar regions have the possibility of neutral and non-neutral positioning. Mitchell[2] summarizes Fryette's Laws as follows:

Fryette's Laws

- **Law 1.** Neutral sidebending produces rotation to the other side or, in other words, the sidebending group rotates itself toward the convexity of the sidebend, with maximum rotation at the apex.

- **Law 2.** Non-neutral (vertebra hyperflexed or hyperextended) rotation and sidebending go to the same side, individual joints acting at one time.
- **Law 3.** Introducing motion to a vertebral joint in one plane automatically reduces its mobility in the other two planes.

Research into coupled movement has been undertaken on cadavers and live subjects. Cadaver research has allowed precise measurements to be taken of coupling behaviour, but has the disadvantage of being unable to reflect the activity of muscles or the accurate effects of load on different postures. Plain radiography has been superseded by the more accurate biplanar radiographic studies that allow research to be undertaken under more normal physiological conditions. Most research has been performed on the lumbar spine.

Reviews of the literature conclude that coupled motion exists but there is conflicting evidence as to the specific characteristics of coupled motion.[11–14] Many authors have demonstrated a coupling relationship between sideflexion and rotation[8,15–29] but there is inconsistent reporting of the direction of coupling.[30] Other authors maintain that sidebending and rotation are purely uniplanar motion occurring independently of each other.[31,32]

Cervical spine (Fig. 3.4)

Stoddard[15] demonstrated radiologically that sidebending in the cervical spine is always accompanied by rotation to the same side regardless of cervical posture. Stoddard's observations in relation to the cervical spine are consistent with Lovett's findings and Fryette's Laws. These findings are further supported by research undertaken using biplanar X-ray analysis[20] and stereophotogrammetry.[24] In 20 normal male volunteers, when the head was rotated, lateral bending occurred by coupling in the same direction at each segment below the C3 vertebra. Interestingly coupling was not restricted to lateral bending. At the same time, flexion took place by coupling at each segment below the C5–6 vertebra and extension above the C4–5 level. In a study of active range of motion in the cervical spine during daily functional tasks, Bennett et al[25] noted that the normal coupling pattern for the cervical spine is rotation and sidebending to the same side. Three-dimensional magnetic resonance imaging (MRI) confirms that the coupling of lateral bending and axial rotation was in the same direction in the cervical spine below C2.[27] Malmstrom et al[26] confirmed this coupling behaviour in asymptomatic subjects up to the age of 70 with decreasing coupling in all cardinal planes with increasing age. Elderly subjects (70–79 years of age) exhibited a change in coupling behaviour with rotation being coupled with contralateral lateral flexion.

Craniocervical junction (Fig. 3.5)

The anatomy of the upper cervical spine differs significantly from the cervical spine below C2. Coupling behaviour has been reported in relation to the upper cervical spine[24,33–35] but has not been as extensively investigated as in other regions of the spine. Stereophotogrammetry revealed consistent coupling of axial rotation and lateral bending to the opposite side at C0–1 and C1–2 and vice versa.[24] Three-dimensional MRI confirmed the relationship between axial rotation and lateral bending to the opposite side.[35] This is the reverse of the coupling behaviour in the cervical spine below C2.

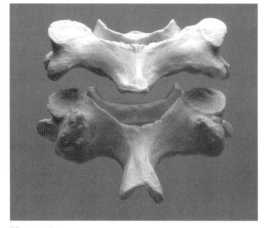

Figure 3.4

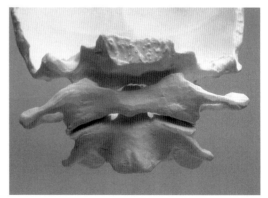

Figure 3.5

Cervicothoracic junction (Fig. 3.6)

There is little information available in relation to the kinematics and coupling behaviour in the junctional region between the flexible cervical spine and the more rigid thoracic region. Osteopathic texts indicate that the prevailing view in relation to coupling in this region is that from C2 to C7 the coupling of axial rotation and lateral flexion is to the same side, whilst below C7 the coupling of axial rotation and lateral flexion can be either to the same or to the opposite side.[9,36]

Computerized tomography (CT) imaging has identified that the cervicothoracic junction is twice as stiff as the rest of the cervical spine. Reliable quantitative data for coupling behaviour of axial rotation and lateral flexion in the cervicothoracic spine remains unreported.[37]

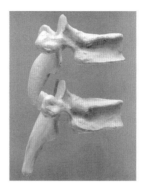

Figure 3.7

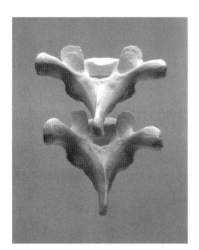

Figure 3.6

Thoracic spine (Fig. 3.7) and lumbar spine (Fig. 3.8)

Although there is agreement as to the direction of axial rotation and lateral flexion coupling in the cervical spine below C2 (i.e. sidebending and rotation occurring to the same side), the patterns for coupling in the lumbar spine are less clear. Stoddard's findings in the lumbar

spine were that 'sidebending is accompanied by rotation to the opposite side if the commencing position is an erect one of extension. If, however, the starting position is full flexion, sidebending is then accompanied by rotation to the same side'.[15] Russell et al, in a study of the range and coupled movements of the lumbar spine using a 3Space Isotrak system on 181 asymptomatic volunteers aged between 20 to 69 years, found that in the erect position there was strong coupling of opposite axial rotation on lateral bending.[23] Despite subjects being told to make lateral flexion as pure a lateral movement as possible, Russell et al also noted a strong coupling of flexion as

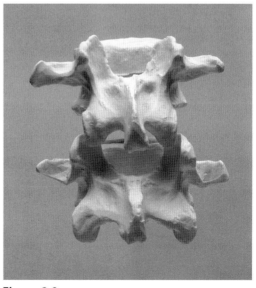

Figure 3.8

17

well as opposite axial rotation on lateral bending. However, other authors do not support these findings and report inconsistent coupling. [8,14,17,19,21,28]

Plamondon et al, using a stereoradiographic method to study lumbar intervertebral motion in vivo, demonstrated that axial rotation and lateral bending were coupled motions but reported there was 'no strict pattern that the vertebra follow in executing a movement'. [19]

Pearcy and Tibrewal, in a three-dimensional radiographic study of normal volunteers with no history of back pain requiring time off work or medical treatment, found that the relationship between axial rotation and lateral bending is not consistent at different levels of the lumbar spine. [17] Some individuals occasionally demonstrate 'movements in the opposite direction to the voluntary movement at individual intervertebral levels, most commonly at L4–5 and L5–S1. In lateral bending, there was a general tendency for L5–S1 to bend in the opposite direction to the voluntary movement.' This unexpected finding is consistent with a study by Weitz. [38]

Panjabi et al, using fresh human cadaveric lumbar spines from L1 to the sacrum, assessed coupled motion under load in different spinal postures using stereophotogrammetry. [21] They concluded that coupling is an inherent property of the lumbar spine as advocated by Lovett [4] but in vitro coupling patterns are more complex than generally believed. They demonstrated the presence of muscles is not a requirement for coupled motion, but acknowledged that they may significantly alter coupling behaviour. The specific effect of physiological loading and muscle activity upon coupled motion is presently unknown. In a neutral posture, left axial torque produced right lateral bending at the upper lumbar levels and left lateral bending at the lower two levels, with L3–4 being a transition level. They concluded that the 'rotary coupling patterns in the lumbar spine are a function of the intervertebral level and posture'. At the upper lumbar levels, axial torque produced lateral bending to the opposite side, whereas at the

lower lumbar levels axial torque produced lateral bending to the same side. It was also noted 'that the spine does not exhibit mechanical reciprocity', for example at L4–5 applied left axial torque produced coupled left lateral bending but applied left lateral bending produced coupled right axial rotation.

The finding of Panjabi et al [21] that at 'L2–3, coupled lateral bending increased from about 0.5° in the fully extended posture to 1.5° in neutral and to about 2° in flexed postures' conflicts with Fryette's Third Law, which indicates that introduction of motion to a vertebral joint in one plane automatically reduces its mobility in the other two planes. In lumbar flexion the coupled lateral bending increased by 0.5° from the neutral to the flexed position.

A number of studies have indicated that coupled movement occurs independently of muscular activity. [8,16,39] In 1977, Pope et al [16] utilized a biplanar radiographic technique to evaluate spinal movements in intact cadaveric and living human subjects. They confirmed that 'vertebral motion occurs as a coupling motion, and that axial rotation uniformly is associated with lateral bend'. Frymoyer et al [39] measured spinal mobility using orthogonal radiography on 20 male cadavers and nine male living subjects. They found that complex coupling does occur in the lumbar spine and demonstrated remarkably similar spinal behaviour between the two groups. These studies indicate that coupling occurs independently of muscular activity.

Vicenzino and Twomey [8] used four human male post-mortem lumbar spines from L1 to the sacrum, with ligaments intact and muscles removed, to assess conjunct rotation of the spine when sidebending was introduced in both a flexed and extended position. They found that, in the flexed position, lateral flexion of the lumbar spine was associated with conjunct rotation to the same side. This is consistent with Fryette's Laws. However, in the extended position, lateral flexion was associated with conjunct rotation to the opposite side, which supports Stoddard's radiographic observations of coupled motion in the extended position. [15] These findings are not consistent with Fryette's Laws, which predict sidebending and rotation to the same side as the facets are not 'idling' when in the extended position. Vicenzino and Twomey's study reveals that the L5–S1 segment is unique in that conjunct rotation was always in the same direction as sideflexion, independent of flexion or extension positioning.[8] This finding for the L5–S1 segment was supported by Pearcy and Tibrewal, who found that, during axial rotation at L5–S1, lateral bending always occurred in the same direction as the axial rotation.[17]

Vicenzino and Twomey[8] draw the conclusion that, as both in vitro and in vivo studies have demonstrated conjunct rotation, the non-contractile components of the lumbar spine may have primary responsibility for the direction of conjunct rotation and that neuromuscular activity may only modify the coupling. The impact of muscular activity on coupled motion in both the normal and dysfunctional intervertebral joint requires further study.

The presence of apophysial joint tropism might influence spinal motion and confound predictive models of vertebral coupling. The incidence of facet tropism has been reported as 20% at all lumbar levels but may increase to 30% at the L5–S1 segment.[3] The incidence of facet tropism is also higher in patient populations attending manual medicine practitioners. It has been estimated that as many as 90% of patients presenting with low back pain and sciatica have articular tropism with pain occurring on the side of the more obliquely oriented facet.[3] Cyron and Hutton[40] subjected 23 cadaveric lumbar intervertebral joints to a combination of compressive and shear forces. When asymmetric facets were present, the vertebrae that have such facets rotated towards the side of the more oblique facet. They concluded articular tropism could lead to lumbar instability manifesting itself as joint rotation toward the side of the more oblique facet. This was not a study of coupled motion and no clear comments can therefore be made about the influence of facet tropism on patterns of coupling but it does suggest that tropism can influence spinal mechanics.

Disc degeneration and spinal pathology presenting with pain and nerve root signs might also influence spinal coupling. In 1985, Pearcy et al[18] undertook a three-dimensional radiographic analysis of lumbar spinal movements. They studied patients with back pain alone and patients with back pain plus nerve tension signs demonstrated by restricted straight leg raise. Coupled movements were increased only in those patients without nerve tension signs indicating the possibility of asymmetrical muscle action. It was concluded that 'the disturbance from the normal pattern of coupled movements in the group with back pain alone suggests that the ligaments or muscles were involved unilaterally and thus acted asymmetrically when the patient moved'. The fact that coupled movements were increased in the back pain group suggests that muscular activity, while not being essential for coupling, can influence the magnitude of coupled movement. The action of the contractile elements in normal, dysfunctional and pain states requires more study before any definite statements can be made relating to their effect upon coupled motion. Using percutaneous transpedicular screws and optoelectronic camera measurement, Lund et al demonstrated that chronic low back pain patients had different coupling behaviour from that of the normal population.[41]

It is evident that many factors, such as facet tropism, vertebral level, intervertebral disc height, back pain and spinal position, might influence the degree and direction of coupling.

Although it appears that Fryette's Laws are open to question and clinicians' concepts of lumbar coupling are inconsistent,[42] there are still only two possibilities for the coupling of sidebending and rotation: to the same or the opposite side. With this in mind, it appears reasonable to classify spinal movement as Type 1 and Type 2 in relation to coupled sidebending and rotation. What is not clearly established is the influence of flexion and extension in relation to Type 1 and Type 2 movements.

CONCLUSION

Conclusions that can be drawn from the literature are limited for a number of reasons. Cadaver studies exclude the effects of muscular activity and normal physiological loading; the studies were also often single segment analysis and generally of small sample size. Plain radiographic studies have inherent measuring difficulties associated with extrapolating three-dimensional movements from two-dimensional films. The use of biplanar radiographic assessment, CT and MRI improved the accuracy of measurement and allowed studies to be performed with muscular activity and in more normal physiological conditions; again, however, the groups studied were small. Notwithstanding these observations, there are a number of conclusions that can be drawn:

1. Coupled motion occurs in all regions of the spine.
2. Coupled motion occurs independently of muscular activity but muscular activity might influence the direction and magnitude of coupled movement.
3. Coupling of sidebending and rotation in the thoracic and lumbar spine is variable in degree and direction.
4. Many variables can influence the degree and direction of coupled movement and include pain, vertebral level, posture and facet tropism.
5. There does not appear to be any simple and consistent relationship between conjunct rotation and intervertebral motion segment level in the thoracic and lumbar spine.

There is evidence to support Lovett's initial observations and Fryette's Laws in relation to sidebending and rotation coupling in the cervical spine, that is, sidebending and rotation occur to the same side.[15,20,24–27] However, the evidence in relation to lumbar and thoracic spine coupling is inconsistent.[8,14,17,19,21,28] Although Fryette's Laws may be useful for predicting coupling behaviour in the cervical spine, caution should be exercised when applying these laws for assessment and treatment of the thoracic and lumbar spine. There has been limited investigation of the coupling behaviour in the craniocervical and cervicothoracic regions. However, evidence suggests that at C0–1 and C1–2 axial rotation and lateral bending occur to opposite sides.[24,35]

References

1 Fryette H. Principles of Osteopathic Technic. Newark, OH: American Academy of Osteopathy; 1954: (Reprint 1990).

2 Mitchell FL. The Muscle Energy Manual. East Lansing, MI: MET Press; 1995.

3 Bogduk N, Twomey LT. Clinical Anatomy of the Lumbar Spine and Sacrum, 3rd edn. Melbourne: Churchill Livingstone; 1997.

4 Lovett RW. The mechanism of the normal spine and its relation to scoliosis. Boston Med Surg J 1905;13:349–358.

5 White A, Panjabi M. Clinical Biomechanics of the Spine. Toronto: Lippincott Company; 1990.

6 Stokes I, Wilder D, Frymoyer J, Pope M. Assessment of patients with low-back pain by biplanar radiographic measurement of intervertebral motion. Spine 1981;6(3):233–240.

7 MacConaill M. The geometry and algebra of articular kinematics. Bio Med Eng 1966;5:205–211.

8 Vicenzino G, Twomey L. Sideflexion induced lumbar spine conjunct rotation and its influencing factors. Aust Physiother 1993;39(4):299–306.

9 Greenman PE. Principles of Manual Medicine, 3rd edn. Philadelphia, PA: Lippincott Williams & Wilkins; 2003.

10 Gibbons P, Tehan P. Muscle energy concepts and coupled motion of the spine. Man Ther 1998;3 (2):95–101.

11 Brown L. An introduction to the treatment and examination of the spine by combined movements. Physiotherapy 1988;74(7):347–353.

12 Brown L. Treatment and examination of the spine by combined movements – 2. Physiotherapy 1990;76(2):666–674.

13 Legaspi O, Edmond S. Does the evidence support the existence of lumbar spine coupled motion? A critical review of the literature. J Orthop & Sports Phys Ther 2007;37(4):169–178.

14 Sizer P, Brismee J-M, Cook C. Coupling behaviour of the thoracic spine: A systematic review of

literature. J Manipulative Physiol Ther 2007;30 (5):390–399.

15 Stoddard A. Manual of Osteopathic Practice. London: Hutchinson Medical Publications; 1969.

16 Pope M, Wilder D, Matteri R, et al. Experimental measurements of vertebral motion under load. Orthop Clin North Am 1977;8(1):155–167.

17 Pearcy M, Tibrewal S. Axial rotation and lateral bending in the normal lumbar spine measured by three-dimensional radiography. Spine 1984;9 (6):582–587.

18 Pearcy M, Portek I, Shepherd J. The effect of low back pain on lumbar spinal movements measured by three-dimensional X-ray analysis. Spine 1985;10 (2):150–153.

19 Plamondon A, Gagnon M, Maurais G. Application of a stereoradiographic method for the study of intervertebral motion. Spine 1988;13(9): 1027–1032.

20 Mimura M, Moriya H, Watanabe T, et al. Three dimensional motion analysis of the cervical spine with special reference to the axial rotation. Spine 1989;14(11):1135–1139.

21 Panjabi M, Yamamoto I, Oxland T, et al. How does posture affect coupling in the lumbar spine? Spine 1989;14(9):1002–1011.

22 Nagerl H, Kubein-Meesenburg D, Fanghanel J. Elements of a general theory of joints. Anat Anz 1992;174(1):66–75.

23 Russell P, Pearcy M, Unsworth A. Measurement of the range and coupled movements observed in the lumbar spine. Br J Rheumatol 1993;32(6): 490–497.

24 Panjabi M, Crisco J, Vasavada A, et al. Mechanical properties of the human cervical spine as shown by three-dimensional load–displacement curves. Spine 2001;26(24):2692–2700.

25 Bennett SE, Schenk R, Simmons E. Active range of motion utilized in the cervical spine to perform daily functional tasks. J Spinal Disord Tech 2002;15(4):307–311.

26 Malmstrom E-M, Karlberg M, Fransson P, et al. Primary and coupled cervical movements. The effect of age, gender, and body mass index. A 3-dimensional movement analysis of a population without symptoms of neck disorders. Spine 2006;31(2):E44–E50.

27 Ishii T, Mukai Y, Hosono N, et al. Kinematics of the cervical spine in lateral bending. In vivo three-dimensional analysis. Spine 2006;31 (2):155–160.

28 Edmondston S, Aggerholm M, Elfving S, et al. Influence of posture on the range of axial rotation and coupled lateral flexion of the thoracic spine. J Manipulative Physiol Ther 2007;30(3):193–199.

29 Fujii R, Sakaura H, Mukai Y, et al. Kinematics of the lumbar spine in trunk rotation: In vivo three-dimensional analysis using magnetic resonance imaging. Eur Spine J 2007;16 (11):1867–1874.

30 Cook C. Coupling behavior of the lumbar spine: A literature review. J Man Manipulative Ther 2003;11 (3):137–145.

31 Schultz A, Warwick D, Berkson M, et al. Mechanical properties of human lumbar spine motion segments – Part 1. J Biomechanical Eng 1979;101:46–52.

32 McGlashen K, Miller A, Schultz A, et al. Load displacement behaviour of the human lumbo-sacral joint. J Orthop Res 1987;5:488–496.

33 Panjabi M, Oda T, Crisco J, et al. Posture affects motion coupling patterns of the upper cervical spine. J Orthop Res 1993;11(4):525–536.

34 Amiri M, Jull G, Bullock-Saxton J. Measurement of upper cervical flexion and extension with the 3-space fastrack measurement system: A repeatability study. J Man Manipulative Ther 2003;11 (4):198–203.

35 Ishii T, Mukai Y, Hosono N, et al. Kinematics of the upper cervical spine in rotation. In vivo three-dimensional analysis. Spine 2004;29(7): E139–E144.

36 Kuchera M. Examination and Diagnosis: An introduction. In: Ward R ed. Foundations for Osteopathic Medicine. Philadelphia: Lippincott Williams & Wilkins; 1997: Ch. 43.

37 Simon S, Davis M, Odhner D, et al. CT imaging techniques for describing motions of the cervicothoracic junction and cervical spine during flexion, extension, and cervical traction. Spine 2006;31(1):44–50.

38 Weitz E. The lateral bending sign. Spine 1981;6 (4):388–397.

39 Frymoyer JW, Frymoyer WW, Wilder DG, et al. The mechanical and kinematic analysis of the lumbar spine in normal living human subjects in vivo. J Biomechanics 1979;12:165–172.

40 Cyron BM, Hutton WC. Articular tropism and stability of the lumbar spine. Spine 1980;5 (2):168–172.

41 Lund T, Nydegger T, Ing D, et al. Three-dimensional motion patterns during active bending in patients with chronic low back pain. Spine 2002;27(17):1865–1874.

42 Cook C, Showalter C. A survey on the importance of lumbar coupling biomechanics in physiotherapy practice. Man Ther 2004;9(3):164–172.

4

Spinal positioning and locking

Note: Principles of spinal positioning & locking on the DVD-ROM should be viewed in conjunction with Chapter 4.

SPINAL LOCKING

Spinal locking is necessary for long-lever high-velocity low-amplitude (HVLA) thrust techniques to localize forces and achieve cavitation at a specific vertebral segment.[1-7] Short-lever HVLA thrust techniques do not require locking of adjacent spinal segments.

Locking can be achieved by either facet apposition or the utilization of ligamentous myofascial tension, or a combination of both.[1-5,7] The principle used in these approaches is to position the spine in such a way that leverage is localized to one joint without undue strain being placed upon adjacent segments.

The osteopathic profession developed a nomenclature to classify spinal motion based upon the coupling of sidebending and rotation movements. This coupling behaviour will vary depending upon spinal positioning:

- **Type 1 movement** – sidebending and rotation occur in opposite directions (Fig. 4.1[8])
- **Type 2 movement** – sidebending and rotation occur in the same direction (Fig. 4.2[8]).

The principle of facet apposition locking is to apply leverages to the spine that cause the facet joints of uninvolved segments to be apposed and consequently locked. To achieve locking by facet apposition, the spine is placed in a position opposite to that of normal coupling behaviour. The vertebral segment at which you wish to produce cavitation should never be locked.

SPINAL POSITIONING

When applying HVLA thrust techniques, it is important to understand that the model presented relates to spinal positioning and locking and is not a model for evaluation and diagnosis of somatic dysfunction.

Cervical spine

A number of authors describe the normal coupling at the occipito-atlantal (C0–1) segment as axial rotation and lateral bending to the opposite side (i.e. Type 1 movement).[7,9,10] The principle of facet apposition locking does not apply to HVLA thrust techniques directed to the C0–1 segment. However, facet apposition locking of the C0–1 segment can be utilized for HVLA thrust techniques directed to other cervical levels (Table 4.1).

The type of coupled movement available at the C1–2 segment is complex. This segment has a predominant role in total cervical rotation.[11-14] Up to 77% of total cervical rotation occurs at the atlanto-axial joint, with a mean rotation range of 40.5° to either side.[11,13] The great range of rotation at the atlanto-axial joint can be attributed to facet plane, the loose nature of the ligamentous fibrous capsule and the absence of ligamentum flavum above C2.[14] Only a small amount of rotation occurs at the joints above and below the atlanto-axial joint.[15-17]

Below C2, normal coupling behaviour in the cervical spine is Type 2 (i.e. sidebending and rotation occur to the same side).[7,9,18-22]

23

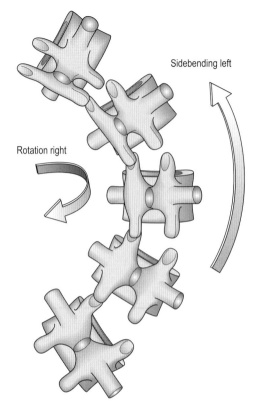

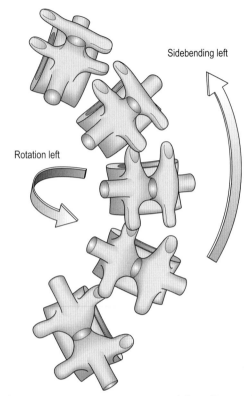

Figure 4.1 Type 1 movement. Sidebending and rotation occur to opposite sides.
(Reproduced with permission from Gibbons and Tehan.[8])

Figure 4.2 Type 2 movement. Sidebending and rotation occur to the same side.
(Reproduced with permission from Gibbons and Tehan.[8])

Table 4.1

Spinal level	Coupled motion	Facet apposition locking
C0–1 (occipito-atlantal)	Type 1	Type 2
C1–2 (atlanto-axial)	Complex-primary rotation	Not Applicable
C2–7	Type 2	Type 1

The average range of cervical spine rotation from neutral position is 80° (Fig. 4.3).[23] For patient comfort and safety the practitioner should limit the total range of cervical spine rotation when applying thrust techniques. Below C2 this is achieved by combining cervical spine rotation with opposite sidebending (Fig. 4.4). To generate facet apposition locking for HVLA thrust techniques, the operator must introduce a Type 1 movement, which is sidebending of

the cervical spine in one direction and rotation in the opposite direction (e.g. sidebending right with rotation left). This positioning locks the segments above the joint to be cavitated and enables a thrust to be applied to one vertebral segment. The amount or degree of sidebending and rotation can be varied to obtain facet locking. The intent should be to have a primary and secondary leverage. The principal or primary leverage can be either sidebending or rotation (Fig. 4.5).

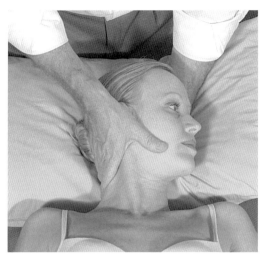

Figure 4.3 Full left cervical spine rotation.

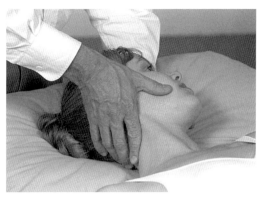

Figure 4.5 Cervical HVLA positioning for up-slope gliding thrust. Primary leverage of rotation to the left and secondary leverage of sidebending to the right achieve facet apposition locking down to the desired segment on the right.

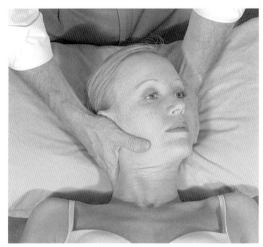

Figure 4.4 Introduction of right sidebending limits the range of available left cervical spine rotation.

The principles of facet apposition locking that apply to the cervical spine are also utilized for HVLA thrust techniques to the cervicothoracic junction (C7–T3). If cervicothoracic region techniques require locking via the cervical spine, this is achieved by introducing Type 1 movements to the cervical spine.

Thoracic and lumbar spine

Current research relating to coupled movements of sidebending and rotation in the thoracic and lumbar spine is inconsistent.

Although research does not validate any single model for spinal positioning and locking in the thoracic and lumbar spine, the model in Table 4.2 is useful for teaching HVLA thrust techniques.

Evidence supports the view that spinal posture and positioning alter coupling behaviour.[24–27] This has implications for joint locking in the thoracic and lumbar spine. In relation to patient positioning, the locking procedures will be different depending on whether the patient's spine is placed in a flexed or a neutral / extended position with evidence indicating that small changes in flexion or extension can significantly alter coupling behaviour.[27]

There is some evidence to support the view that, in the flexed position, the coupling of sidebending and rotation is to the same side,[24–26] whereas in the neutral / extended position the coupling of sidebending and rotation occurs to opposite sides.[24,25,28] The model outlined in Table 4.2 incorporates the available evidence and is useful in the teaching and application of HVLA thrust techniques. Because the evidence for coupling behaviour is inconsistent, it must be understood that this is a model for facet apposition locking which cannot be relied upon in all circumstances.

25

Table 4.2

	Coupled motion	Facet apposition locking
Spinal level		
C7–T3	Type 1 or Type 2	Type 2 or Type 1
T3–L5	Type 1 or Type 2	Type 2 or Type 1
Position of spine T3–L5		
Flexion	Type 2	Type 1 – sidebending and rotation to the opposite side
Neutral / extension	Type 1	Type 2 – sidebending and rotation to the same side

For patient comfort and safety, the practitioner should limit the total amount of trunk rotation when using HVLA thrust techniques in the thoracolumbar and lumbar spine. In most instances, this can be achieved using the facet apposition model and an understanding of coupled motion in the neutral / extension and flexion position prior to the application of a HVLA thrust technique. These techniques can be applied in either a neutral / extension or in a flexed position. In the example of neutral / extension positioning (Fig. 4.6), the practitioner uses spinal positioning and locking to limit the total range of trunk rotation. If the practitioner introduces trunk flexion from below (Fig. 4.7), or from above and below (Fig. 4.8), an increased range of trunk rotation is then required to achieve the necessary locking prior to the application of an HVLA thrust technique.

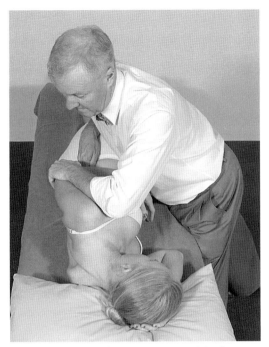

Figure 4.6 Neutral / extension positioning.

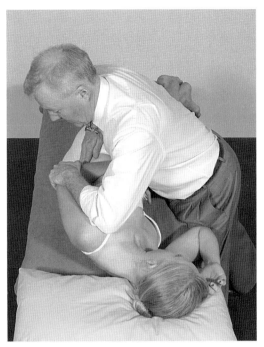

Figure 4.8 Note further increased rotation necessary to achieve locking with introduction of trunk flexion from both above and below.

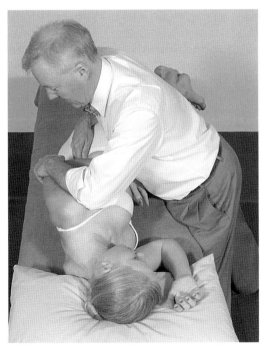

Figure 4.7 Note increased rotation necessary to achieve locking with introduction of trunk flexion from below.

27

Neutral / extension positioning

The patient's lumbar and thoracic spine is positioned in a neutral / extended posture (Fig. 4.9). Using the model outlined, the normal coupling behaviour of sidebending and rotation in the neutral / extension position is Type 1 movement. Facet apposition locking will be achieved by introducing a Type 2 movement (i.e. sidebending and rotation to the same side).

The spine in the neutral / extension position is slung between the pelvis and shoulder girdle and creates a long C curve with the trunk sidebending to the patient's right when the patient lies on the left side.

Trunk rotation to the right is introduced by gently pushing the patient's upper shoulder away from the operator. Rotation and sidebending to the same side achieve facet apposition locking in the neutral or extended position, in this instance with sidebending and rotation to the right (Fig. 4.10).

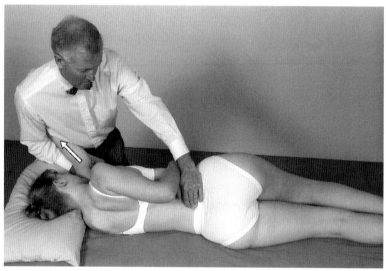

Figure 4.9 Neutral / extension positioning. ⇨ Direction of body movement (patient).

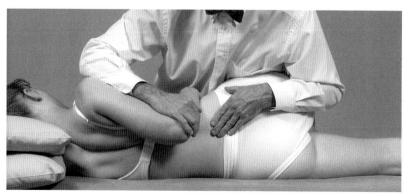

Figure 4.10 Neutral / extension positioning. Type 2 locking. Rotation and sidebending to the same side, i.e. sidebending right and rotation right.

Flexion positioning

The patient's lumbar and thoracic spine is positioned in a flexed posture (Fig. 4.11). The normal coupling behaviour of sidebending and rotation in the flexed position is Type 2 movement. Facet apposition locking will be achieved by introducing a Type 1 movement (i.e. sidebending and rotation to opposite sides).

To achieve facet apposition locking of the spine, in the flexed posture, the trunk must be rotated and sidebent to opposite sides. The operator introduces trunk sidebending to the left by placing a rolled towel under the patient's thoracolumbar spine. Trunk rotation to the right is introduced by gently pushing the patient's upper shoulder away from the operator (Fig. 4.12).

Many factors, such as facet tropism, vertebral level, intervertebral disc height, back pain and spinal position, can affect coupling behaviour and there will be occasions when the model outlined needs to be modified to suit an individual patient. In such circumstances, the operator will need to adjust patient positioning to facilitate effective localization of forces. To achieve this, the operator must develop the palpatory skills necessary to sense appropriate pre-thrust tension and leverage prior to delivering the HVLA thrust.

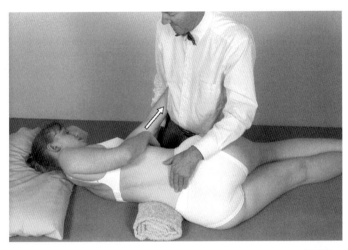

Figure 4.11 Flexion positioning. ⇨ Direction of body movement (patient).

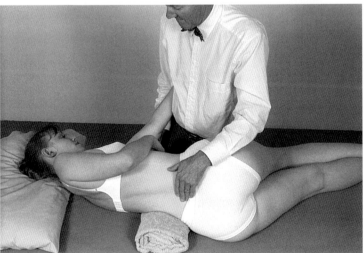

Figure 4.12 Flexion positioning. Type 1 locking. Rotation and sidebending to opposite sides, i.e. sidebending left and rotation right.

RATIONALE FOR CHOICE OF POSITIONING

The rationale underpinning patient positioning when applying HVLA thrust techniques is to use a model of coupling behaviour that facilitates effective localization of forces to a specific segment of the spine prior to the application of a thrust. The joint to be thrust should not be locked by facet apposition but remain free. Patient comfort is the criterion for selecting either the neutral / extension or flexion positioning in the thoracic and lumbar spine techniques – that is, the most comfortable position for the patient to assume prior to the delivery of the thrust.

References

1 Nyberg R. Manipulation: definition, types, application. In: Basmajian J, Nyberg R eds. 1993. Rational Manual Therapies. Baltimore, MD: Williams & Wilkins; 1993:21–47.

2 Downing CH. Principles and Practice of Osteopathy. London: Tamor Pierston; 1985.

3 Stoddard A. Manual of Osteopathic Technique, 2nd edn. London: Hutchinson Medical; 1972.

4 Hartman L. Handbook of Osteopathic Technique, 3rd edn. London: Chapman & Hall; 1997.

5 Beal MC. Teaching of basic principles of osteopathic manipulative techniques. In: Beal M C ed. 1989. The Principles of Palpatory Diagnosis and Manipulative Technique. Newark: American Academy of Osteopathy; 1989:162–164.

6 Kappler RE. Direct action techniques. In: Beal M C ed. 1989. The Principles of Palpatory Diagnosis and Manipulative Technique. Newark: American Academy of Osteopathy; 1989:165–168.

7 Greenman PE. Principles of Manual Medicine, 3rd edn. Philadelphia, PA: Lippincott Williams & Wilkins; 2003.

8 Gibbons P, Tehan P. Muscle energy concepts and coupled motion of the spine. Man Ther 1998;3 (2):95–101.

9 Panjabi M, Crisco J, Vasavada A, et al. Mechanical properties of the human cervical spine as shown by three-dimensional load–displacement curves. Spine 2001;26 (24):2692–2700.

10 Ishii T, Mukai Y, Hosono N, et al. Kinematics of the upper cervical spine in rotation. In vivo three-dimensional analysis. Spine 2004;29(7): E139–E144.

11 Penning L, Wilmink JT. Rotation of the cervical spine: a CT study in normal subjects. Spine 1987;12(8):732–738.

12 Mimura M, Moriya H, Watanabe T, et al. Three dimensional motion analysis of the cervical spine with special reference to axial rotation. Spine 1989;14(11):1135–1139.

13 Iai H, Moriya H, Takahashi K, et al. Three dimensional motion analysis of upper cervical spine during axial rotation. Spine 1993;18 (16):2388–2392.

14 Guth M. A comparison of cervical rotation in age-matched adolescent competitive swimmers and healthy males. J Orthop Sports Phys Ther 1995;21 (1):21–27.

15 Penning L. Normal movements of the cervical spine. J Roentgenol 1978;130(2):317–326.

16 White A, Panjabi M. Clinical Biomechanics of the Spine, 2nd edn. Philadelphia, PA: Lippincott; 1990.

17 Porterfield JA, DeRosa C. Mechanical Neck Pain: Perspectives in Functional Anatomy. Sydney: WB Saunders; 1995.

18 Mimura M, Moriya H, Watanabe T, et al. Three dimensional motion analysis of the cervical spine with special reference to the axial rotation. Spine 1989;14(11):1135–1139.

19 Stoddard A. Manual of Osteopathic Practice. London: Hutchinson Medical; 1969.

20 Bennett SE, Schenk R, Simmons E. Active range of motion utilized in the cervical spine to perform daily functional tasks. J Spinal Disord Tech 2002;15(4):307–311.

21 Ishii T, Mukai Y, Hosono N, et al. Kinematics of the cervical spine in lateral bending. In vivo three-dimensional analysis. Spine 2006;31 (2):155–160.

22 Malmstrom E-M, Karlberg M, Fransson P, et al. Primary and coupled cervical movements. The effect of age, gender, and body mass index. A 3-Dimensional movement analysis of a population without symptoms of neck disorders. Spine 2006;31(2):E44–E50.

23 American Medical Association. Guides to the Evaluation of Permanent Impairment, 4th edn. Chicago, IL: American Medical Association; 1999.

24 Vicenzino G, Twomey L. Sideflexion induced lumbar spine conjunct rotation and its influencing factors. Aust Physiother 1993;39 (4):299–306.

25 Fryette H. Principles of Osteopathic Technic. Newark, OH: American Academy of Osteopathy; 1954:'15–21:(reprinted 1990).

26 Panjabi M, Yamamoto I, Oxland T, et al. How does posture affect coupling in the lumbar spine? Spine 1989;14(9):1002–1011.

27 Drake J, Callaghan J. Do flexion / extension postures affect the in vivo passive lumbar spine response to applied axial twist moments? Clin Biomechanics 2008;23 (5):510–519.

28 Russell P, Pearcy M, Unsworth A. Measurement of the range and coupled movements observed in the lumbar spine. Br J Rheumatol 1993;32 (6):490–497.

5

Safety and HVLA thrust techniques

INTRODUCTION

There are risks and benefits associated with any therapeutic intervention. High-velocity low-amplitude (HVLA) thrust techniques are distinguished from other osteopathic techniques because the practitioner applies a rapid thrust or impulse. Thrust or impulse techniques are considered to be potentially more dangerous when compared with non-impulse mobilization.

COMPLICATIONS

Incidence

Most published literature relating to the incidence of injury resulting from manipulative techniques focuses upon serious sequelae resulting from cervical spine manipulation.

There is wide variation in estimated serious adverse reactions arising from cervical manipulation. Various authors have attempted to estimate the incidence of iatrogenic stroke following cervical spine manipulation.[1-14] Estimates vary from one incident in 10 000 cervical spine manipulations to one incident in 5.85 million cervical spine manipulations. Rivett and Milburn[12] estimated the incidence of severe neurovascular compromise to be within the range one in 50 000 to one in 5 million cervical spine manipulations. Other authors estimate complications for cervical spine manipulation to be 1.46 times per 1 million manipulations[15] and 1 case of cerebrovascular accident in every 1.3 million cervical

treatment sessions increasing to one in every 0.9 million for upper cervical manipulation.[9] Dvorak and Orelli[3] report a rate of one serious complication per 400 000 cervical manipulations while Patijn[11] found an overall rate of one complication per 518 886 manipulations. Miley et al[14] estimated the incidence of vertebral artery dissection attributable to cervical spine manipulation as 1.3 cases for every 100 000 persons less than 45 years of age within 1 week of manipulation. The published research does not make clear which types of neck manipulation technique were applied, or the competence and training of the practitioner.[16]

Published figures may not accurately reflect the true incidence of serious cervical spine complications.[10-12,17-19] The frequency with which complications arise in patients receiving cervical spine manipulation can only be an estimate as the true number of manipulations performed and the numbers of patients receiving cervical manipulation remain unknown.[20] In relation to vertebral artery dissection, Haldeman et al[21] indicate that a database of multiple millions of cervical manipulations are necessary to obtain accurate statistics. Such a complication can arise from normal neck movements and trivial trauma and not only from cervical manipulation.[21-28] Haldeman et al[21] reviewed the published literature to assess the risk factors and precipitating neck movements causing vertebrobasilar artery dissection. A total of 367 cases were identified, of which 252 were either of spontaneous onset, or related to trivial (Table 5.1) or major trauma.

33

Table 5.1 Description of trivial trauma associated with vertebrobasilar artery dissection / occlusion cases

Type of trivial trauma	Examples	No. of cases
Sporting activities	Basketball, tennis, softball, swimming, callisthenics	18
Leisure activities	Walking, kneeling at prayer, household chores, sexual intercourse	8
Sustained rotation and / or extension	Wallpapering, washing walls and ceilings, archery, yoga	10
Short-lived rotation and / or extension	Turning head while driving, backing out of driveway, looking up	7
Sudden head movements	Sneezing, fair ride, violent coughing, sudden head flexion	7
Miscellaneous, minor trauma	Minor fall, 'banging' head	2
Miscellaneous	Atlanto-axial instability, postpartum, post gastrectomy	6
Total		58

Haldeman et al.[21]

Less than one-third of cases (115) were associated with cervical manipulation.[21] Haneline and Lewkovich[23] undertook a literature search of the MEDLINE database for published articles relating to cervical artery dissection between 1994 and 2003. Twenty studies met the selection criteria reporting 606 cervical artery dissection cases. The authors concluded that a minority of cases was associated with cervical spine manipulation. A summary of the findings is outlined in Box 5.1.

Difficulties arise in the estimation of risk for vertebrobasilar dissection after neck manipulation, as patients may in fact seek treatment for symptoms of a progressing dissection.[28] Smith et al[29] attempted to address this issue in a case controlled study of the association between neck manipulation and cervical arterial dissection and reported that neck manipulation is an independent risk factor for vertebral artery dissection even after controlling for neck pain. A population-based, case control and case crossover study identified that primary care physician visits and attendance for chiropractic treatment for headache and neck pain were both strongly associated with subsequent vertebrobasilar artery stroke when compared with age- and gender-matched controls.[28] This raises the possibility that patients with a symptomatic vertebral artery dissection seek clinical care prior to progressing to a vertebrobasilar stroke. Williams et al[30] indicate that estimates for stroke following neck manipulation will always be difficult to quantify. Selection, referral and recall bias in addition to age-related variables have the potential to confound estimation of the risk of vertebrobasilar dissection after neck manipulation.[30,31]

The majority of published articles on complications of spinal manipulation have focused upon vascular consequences but non-vascular complications following spinal manipulation have also been documented.[32]

Box 5.1 Aetiology of cervical artery dissections

- 54% internal carotid artery dissection
- 46% vertebral artery dissection
- 61% classified as spontaneous
- 30% associated with trauma / trivial trauma
- 9% associated with cervical spinal manipulation

(Reproduced with permission from Haneline et al.[23])

Serious complications are extremely uncommon and adverse consequences such as worsening lumbar disc herniation or cauda equina syndrome were found to be extremely rare in five systematic reviews of spinal manipulation.[33] A systematic review of 73 randomized clinical trials reported no serious complication from spinal manipulation.[34] A systematic review of the safety of spinal manipulation in the treatment of lumbar disc herniations reported the risk of a patient suffering a clinically worsened disc herniation or cauda equina syndrome following spinal manipulation to be less than 1 in 3.7 million.[35] Although it is recognized that spinal manipulation is not without some risks, Haldeman has commented that it should be considered one of the safest forms of treatment available for spinal disorders.[36]

Classification of complications

Complications can be classified as transient, substantive reversible impairment, substantive non-reversible impairment and serious non-reversible impairment.

Transient

- Local pain or discomfort
- Stiffness
- Headache
- Tiredness / fatigue
- Radiating pain or discomfort

Transient side-effects following cervical spine manipulation are relatively common.[37] Less common transient reactions include dizziness or imbalance, extremity weakness, ringing in the ears, depression or anxiety, nausea or vomiting, blurred or impaired vision, confusion or disorientation.[38]

Transient side-effects resulting from manipulative treatment may be more common than one might expect and may remain unreported by patients unless information is explicitly requested. Prospective studies report common side-effects resulting from spinal

manipulation occur between 30% and 61% of patients.[39–43] These side-effects usually begin within 4 hours and resolve within the next 24 hours.[41]

Substantive reversible impairment

Cervical spine

- Disc herniation / prolapse
- Nerve root compression
- Cervical and upper thoracic spine strain

Thoracic spine

- Minor vertebral body compression fracture
- Posterior element fracture without loss of structural integrity
- Pneumothorax
- Shoulder girdle, thoracic spine and rib cage strain

Lumbar spine

- Minor vertebral body compression fracture
- Posterior element fracture without loss of structural integrity
- Disc herniation / prolapse
- Nerve root compression
- Shoulder girdle, thoracic spine and lumbopelvic region strain

Substantive non-reversible impairment

Cervical spine

- Unresolved disc herniation / prolapse / extrusion
- Unresolved radiculopathy

Thoracic spine

- Significant vertebral body compression fracture
- Posterior element fracture with disruption of the spinal canal

Lumbar spine

- Significant vertebral body compression fracture
- Posterior element fracture with disruption of the spinal canal
- Unresolved disc herniation / prolapse / extrusion
- Unresolved radiculopathy

Serious non-reversible impairment

Cervical spine

- Death
- Cerebrovascular accident
- Spinal cord compression

Thoracic spine

- Spinal cord compression

Lumbar spine

- Cauda equina syndrome

Causes of complications

Complications associated with the use of HVLA thrust techniques generally relate to either incorrect patient selection or poor technique.

Incorrect patient selection

- Lack of diagnosis
- Lack of awareness of possible complications
- Inadequate palpatory assessment
- Lack of patient consent

Poor technique

- Excessive force
- Excessive amplitude
- Excessive leverage
- Inappropriate combination of leverage
- Incorrect plane of thrust
- Poor patient positioning
- Poor operator positioning
- Lack of patient feedback

HVLA THRUST TECHNIQUES AND RELATIVE RISKS

Most of the research and reporting of both transient and more serious complications of manual interventions has focused upon HVLA thrust techniques. The incidence of complications of other manual therapy techniques remains largely unknown. Non-thrust techniques have also been associated with serious adverse consequences. Spontaneous intracranial hypotension has been reported secondary to a dural tear following cervical and thoracic spine mobilization.[44] One case of cerebrovascular accident that only partially recovered and six cases of brachialgia with neurological deficit have been reported following cervical spine mobilization.[45] A case of retinal artery occlusion followed 'low-force joint mobilization from C2 to C7'[46] and cerebral artery embolism has been attributed to Shiatsu massage.[47] An internal carotid dissection followed use of a handheld electric massager.[48] An attitudinal study of Australian Manipulative Physiotherapists who had undertaken specific postgraduate study in manipulative therapy reported that 84.5% used manipulation in the cervical spine and that most adverse effects associated with examination or treatment of the cervical spine arose as a result of passive mobilizing and examination techniques ahead of high-velocity thrust techniques.[49]

Many patients with musculoskeletal conditions are prescribed non-steroidal anti-inflammatory medication. Dabbs and Lauretti[50] reported the incidence of bleeding or perforation following the use of such medication for the treatment of osteoarthritis as being 4 in 1000 patients with death occurring in 4 out of 10 000 patients. The authors conclude that the use of non-steroidal anti-inflammatory medication when compared with cervical manipulation, for the treatment of comparable conditions, poses a significantly greater risk of serious complications and death. A national prospective survey in the United Kingdom of 19 772 patients receiving 50 276 cervical spine manipulations identified that the risk rates of cervical manipulation were comparable to the use of anti-inflammatory medications commonly prescribed for musculoskeletal conditions.[37]

Acupuncture is also used for the treatment of musculoskeletal conditions and is recognized to be a very safe therapeutic intervention in the hands of a competent practitioner.[51] When comparative risk rates are considered those associated with neck manipulation are reported to be lower than those for acupuncture treatment.[37]

Many interventions for the treatment of musculoskeletal conditions are associated with risk but we do not have comparative risk rates compared with HVLA thrust techniques. Myocardial infarction following exercise prescription, allergic reactions to injection therapies, burns from heat, cold and electrotherapy are all well recognized as potential complications.

Even though the documented risk of stroke and death related to cervical spine manipulation appears to be less than other risks encountered in daily life, it is still considered legally pertinent to discuss risk with the patient.[52] If one considers the risk of stroke or death following neck manipulation to be in the mid range of documented figures then the risk is comparable to a patient being involved in a serious plane crash with 0.75 air crashes (hull losses) reported per million departures in 2007.[53] Patients can be informed that they are far more likely to die or be seriously injured in a motor vehicle accident than following cervical spine manipulation.

CONTRAINDICATIONS

Whenever a practitioner applies a therapeutic intervention, due consideration must be given to the risk–benefit ratio. The benefit to the patient must outweigh any potential risk associated with the intervention. Contraindications or red flags can be classified as general or region specific and are identified from the patient's history, physical examination and clinical tests.[54] Contraindications have been classified as absolute and relative. The distinction between absolute and relative contraindications is influenced by factors such as the skill, experience and training of the practitioner, the type of technique selected, the amount of leverage and force used, the age, general health and physique of the patient.

Absolute

- Bone: any pathology that has led to significant bone weakening:
  - Tumour, e.g. metastatic deposits
  - Infection, e.g. tuberculosis
  - Metabolic, e.g. osteomalacia
  - Congenital, e.g. dysplasias
  - Iatrogenic, e.g. long-term corticosteroid medication
  - Inflammatory, e.g. severe rheumatoid arthritis
  - Traumatic, e.g. fracture
- Neurological
  - Cervical myelopathy
  - Cord compression
  - Cauda equina compression
  - Nerve root compression with increasing neurological deficit
- Vascular
  - Diagnosed vertebrobasilar insufficiency
  - Diagnosed carotid artery dysfunction
  - Aortic aneurysm
  - Bleeding diatheses, e.g. severe haemophilia
- Lack of a diagnosis
- Lack of patient consent
- Patient positioning cannot be achieved because of pain or resistance

Relative

Certain categories of patients have an increased potential for adverse reactions following the application of an HVLA thrust technique. Special consideration should be given prior to the use of HVLA thrust technique in the following circumstances:

- Adverse reactions to previous manual therapy
- Disc herniation or prolapse
- Inflammatory arthritides
- Pregnancy
- Spondylolysis
- Spondylolisthesis
- Osteoporosis
- Anticoagulant or long-term corticosteroid use
- Advanced degenerative joint disease and spondylosis
- Vertigo
- Psychological dependence upon HVLA thrust technique
- Ligamentous laxity / hypermobility
- Arterial calcification

The above list is not intended to cover all possible clinical situations. Patients who have pathology may also have coincidental spinal pain and discomfort arising from mechanical dysfunction that may benefit from manipulative treatment.

HVLA THRUST TECHNIQUES AND DISC LESIONS

The diagnosis of disc pathology is achieved by clinical examination and imaging modalities including computerized tomography (CT) and magnetic resonance imaging (MRI) (Fig. 5.1)[55]. A number of studies have reported imaging evidence of a disc abnormality in asymptomatic individuals.[56–62] Another study has reported patients with low back pain and imaging evidence of disc abnormality responding favourably to manipulative treatment without any alteration in the MRI findings.[63] Abnormal disc imaging findings may frequently be coincidental to a patient's symptoms and are not reliable predictors for the presence, development or duration of spinal pain. It has been reported that a high rate of asymptomatic subjects have disc herniation on MRI imaging and that clinicians need to be aware that MRI images are not necessarily a causal explanation of a patient's pain.[62] The diagnosis of discogenic pain

should not be made from imaging findings alone but must also take into account a patient's age, clinical signs and symptoms.

The use of HVLA thrust techniques for patients with disc bulging or herniation is often cited as being controversial but many authors do support the use of manipulation.[63–69]

One study of 27 patients with MRI documented and symptomatic disc herniation of the cervical and lumbar spine reported that 80% of subjects achieved a good clinical outcome, which suggests that chiropractic care including spinal manipulation may be a safe and effective treatment approach for patients presenting with symptomatic cervical or lumbar disc herniation.[66] Other studies have also reported symptomatic benefits associated with spinal manipulation in patients with disc lesions.[63,66,68,69]

A review of the published data on the efficacy of spinal manipulation in the management of disc herniation, including published data on harms, reported that adverse events appear to be rare and manipulation is likely to be safe when used by appropriately trained practitioners.[70] However, there have been case reports of a ruptured cervical disc[71] and lumbar disc

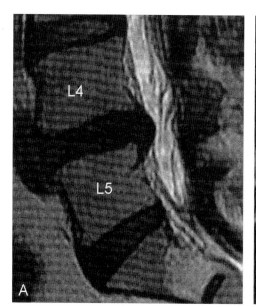
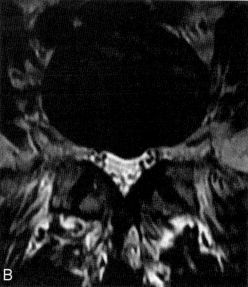

Figure 5.1 L4-5 disc protrusion. A: Sagittal view. B: Axial view. (Reproduced with permission from Elsevier.)[55]

herniation progressing to cauda equina syndrome following manipulative procedures.[72,73] What is not known is whether the disc herniation would have progressed without manipulation or whether the force and torque of the manipulation was a factor. A systematic review of the safety of spinal manipulation in the treatment of lumbar disc herniations reported the risk of a patient suffering a clinically worsened disc herniation or cauda equina syndrome following spinal manipulation to be less than 1 in 3.7 million.[35] A systematic review of HVLA thrust techniques concluded that the evidence does not support the hypothesis that spinal manipulation is inherently unsafe in cases of symptomatic lumbar disc disease.[74]

The use of manipulation techniques under general anaesthesia for low back pain is associated with an increased risk of serious neurological damage.[72] There is no evidence that this approach for the treatment of low back pain is effective.[75]

CERVICAL ARTERY DYSFUNCTION

Adverse events can be associated with compromise of the cervical arterial system. Dissection within the cervical arteries is a recognized cause of ischaemic stroke in the young and middle aged.[76,77] Definitive risk factors for vertebral artery and carotid artery dissection have not been identified. Vascular complications in these vessels can present with neck and head symptoms without the commonly described symptoms associated with vertebrobasilar insufficiency. Cervical artery dissection should always be considered in the differential diagnosis of patients presenting with headache and / or neck pain.[78,79] Both the vertebral and internal carotid arteries should be considered in pre-treatment risk assessment.

The common carotid artery is easily palpable in the neck above the sternocleidomastoid muscle. It divides into the internal and external carotid arteries at the level of the upper border of the thyroid cartilage (Fig. 5.2).[80] The internal carotid artery extends directly upwards and through the base of the skull at the carotid

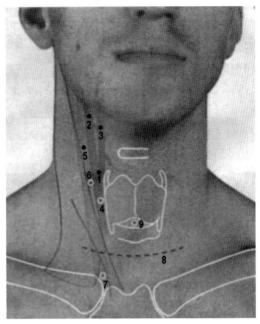

Figure 5.2 Carotid arteries, internal jugular vein and applied anatomy.
1. Common carotid artery
2. Internal carotid artery
3. External carotid artery
4. Point of access to common carotid artery
5. Internal jugular vein
6. Point of access to internal jugular vein above sternocleidomastoid muscle
7. Point of access of internal jugular vein between the heads of the sternocleidomastoid muscle
8. Collar incision
9. Cricothyroid puncture site
(Reproduced with permission from Elsevier.)[80]

canal of the temporal bone to supply the brain. The external carotid artery extends from the bifurcation of the common carotid artery to the neck of the mandible, there dividing into the superficial temporal and maxillary arteries.

The vertebrobasilar system comprises the two vertebral arteries and their union to form the basilar artery (Fig. 5.3). This system supplies approximately 20% of intracranial blood supply.[81] Blood flow in the vertebral artery may be affected by intrinsic and extrinsic factors. Intrinsic factors, such as atherosclerosis, narrow the vessel lumen,

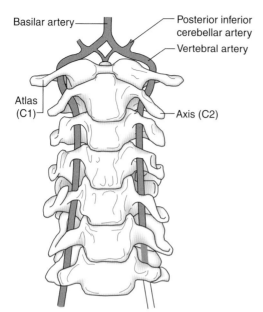

Figure 5.3 Relationship of the cervical spine to the vertebral artery.

increase turbulence and reduce blood flow. Extrinsic factors compress or impinge upon the external wall of the vertebral artery.

There are three areas where the vertebral artery is vulnerable to external compression:

1. At the level of the vertebral foramen of C6 by the contraction of the longus colli and / or the anterior scalene muscles.
2. Within the foramen transversarium between C6 and C2.
3. At the level of C1 and C2 (Fig. 5.4).

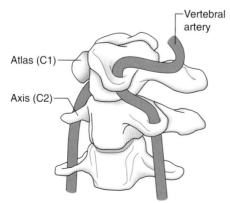

Figure 5.4 Upper cervical rotation stretches the vertebral artery between the atlas and the axis.

VERTEBROBASILAR INSUFFICIENCY

Symptoms and signs of vertebrobasilar insufficiency

The ability to recognize symptoms that may indicate vertebrobasilar insufficiency (VBI) is essential for safe practice. Symptoms of VBI occur because of ischaemia in the structures supplied by the vertebrobasilar system. There are a number of signs and symptoms that may be suggestive of VBI.

Signs of VBI

- Nystagmus
- Gait disturbances
- Horner's syndrome

Symptoms of VBI

- Headache / neck pain (especially if sudden and severe)
- Dizziness / vertigo
- Nausea
- Vomiting
- Diplopia
- Tinnitus
- Drop attacks
- Dysarthria
- Dysphagia
- Facial paraesthesia
- Tingling in the upper limbs
- Pallor and sweating
- Blurred vision
- Light-headedness
- Fainting / blackouts

Diagnosis of VBI

For patients presenting with head and neck pain, especially sudden and severe symptoms, it is important to determine whether there is associated dizziness and / or signs of brain stem ischaemia such as nausea and / or vomiting. Dizziness is also a common presenting complaint with multiple aetiologies that must be distinguished from dizziness arising from VBI (Box 5.2). It has been suggested that questioning about nausea during VBI testing is as important as inquiring

> **Box 5.2** Causes of dizziness
>
> **Systemic causes of dizziness**
> - Medication
> - Hypotension
> - Diabetes
> - Thyroid disease
> - Cardiac or pulmonary insufficiency
>
> **Central causes of dizziness**
> - Demyelinating diseases
> - Tumours of brain or spinal cord
> - Seizures
> - Vertebrobasilar insufficiency
> - Post-traumatic (concussion) vertigo
>
> **Peripheral causes of dizziness**
> - Benign positional vertigo
> - Ménière's disease
> - Cervical spine dysfunction
> - Labyrinthitis
> - Vestibulotoxic medication

about dizziness.[82] Diagnosed VBI is an absolute contraindication to HVLA thrust techniques to the cervical spine.

One difficulty in recognizing the symptoms of VBI is that many of the common symptoms (e.g. headache, pain and stiffness in the cervical spine) are similar to those for mechanical non-specific neck pain.[83,84]

Physical examination

Pre-manipulative testing movements for VBI have been advocated as a means of risk management with a view to minimizing patient harm.[85] There are many physical tests described for determining the presence or absence of VBI.[86–91]

Tests for VBI have been based upon the premise that cervical spine positioning may reduce the lumen and blood flow in the vertebral arteries.[92–97] Studies on cadaveric specimens have demonstrated reduced flow through contralateral vertebral arteries in combined extension and rotation.[98,99] In vivo studies also support the view that cervical spine positioning may reduce vertebral artery blood flow.[94,95,97,100–104] A study of normal volunteers concluded that blood velocity

altered significantly at 45° cervical spine rotation and again at full range cervical spine rotation and in the pre-manipulative position.[94,97] Other studies of vertebral artery blood flow have not identified significant change in flow related to cervical spine positioning.[105–109]

Evidence linking vertebral artery narrowing or occlusion with cervical spine extension and rotation positioning contributed to the development and use of many pre-manipulative tests for VBI. It was postulated that a reduction in blood flow as a result of cervical spine positioning would produce detectable symptoms or signs in a patient with VBI. Positive tests were assumed to be a predictor of patients at risk from cerebrovascular complications of manipulation. However, tests for VBI have poor sensitivity and variable specificity.[110,111] The value of these tests in determining VBI has been questioned.[21,91,112–116]

Research has questioned the continuing role of diagnostic VBI tests. Screening tests should be both valid and reliable predictors of risk. VBI-testing movements have neither of these qualities, with available scientific evidence failing to show predictive value.[20,107,113] Westaway et al[116] report a false-negative VBI test in an asymptomatic subject with a radiographically unstable C1–2 segment and a hypoplastic and atretic right vertebral artery further questioning the predictive value of such screening procedures. Screening procedures should not be harmful. It has been suggested that the tests themselves may hold certain risks and could have a morbid effect on the vertebral artery.[117] Minor adverse effects associated with examination procedures involving rotation, including those related to the use of an established VBI-testing protocol, have been documented.[49]

Symons et al[118] attempted to quantify the internal forces on the vertebral artery during neck manipulation and VBI testing on five unembalmed post-rigor cadavers. Strains sustained internally by the vertebral artery during neck range of motion testing, VBI screening and HVLA thrust techniques were similar and all were significantly less than the forces required to disrupt the vertebral artery mechanically. The study concluded that a single typical HVLA thrust technique to the neck is unlikely to cause mechanical disruption of the vertebral artery.[118]

An analysis of the published literature does not support the continuing use of VBI-screening tests or protocols in isolation as none of the rotation, extension or combination test movements have been shown to be valid or reliable predictors of risk.

Is it possible through physical examination or screening procedures to identify patients at risk of vertebrobasilar injury from cervical spine manipulation? Current evidence would suggest that the answer is no.[6,119–122] A jury in an inquest into the death of a female chiropractic patient following a neck adjustment recommended that:

> Based on evidence heard that practitioners ... be informed by their respective regulatory bodies that provocative testing (prior to performing high neck manipulation) has not been demonstrated to be of benefit and should not be performed. Universities and Colleges teaching high neck manipulation should also be teaching their students that these tests have not been demonstrated to be of benefit and should not be performed.[123]

In the light of current research findings, what would constitute a suitable approach to the pre-manipulative assessment of the cervical spine?

Pre-manipulative assessment

If a significant number of symptoms (e.g. head pain, neck pain, dizziness, nausea and vomiting) are suggestive of cervical artery dysfunction, it would be advisable to proceed with caution when testing full range movement of the cervical spine in patients who present with cervical and cervicothoracic spinal syndromes. Such patients should be referred for the appropriate medical investigation to confirm or rule out the presence of cervical artery dysfunction. The use of HVLA thrust techniques in such patients would be contraindicated until such time as the cause of the symptoms has been clearly established.

If a patient presents with a few symptoms that might be suggestive of cervical artery dysfunction, a normal physical examination would include pain-free range of motion testing of the cervical spine (Figs 5.5–5.10). Such range of motion testing might include both active and passive movements, but would be performed with care and to the point of provocation of symptoms only.

The reports of vascular complications in the literature do not make clear what type of manipulative techniques were associated with vertebral or internal carotid artery complications, nor how well the techniques were applied. The risks associated with HVLA thrust techniques can be minimized by a thorough understanding of spinal locking and positioning procedures as well as the attainment of a high level of psychomotor skill related to the use of minimal leverage, high velocity, low amplitude and controlled manipulative techniques.

The safe application of HVLA thrust techniques is critically linked to comprehensive training and skill development in the appropriateness and delivery of HVLA thrust techniques.

HVLA thrust techniques are believed to carry a higher risk of cervical artery complications than mobilization or non-impulse techniques. This view is challenged by research demonstrating that the strain sustained by the vertebral artery during both the testing of neck range of motion and the application of a single HVLA thrust technique was of a similar magnitude.[118] Practitioners using non-impulse and mobilization techniques also need to be aware that there is a risk of vascular complications with the application of non-thrust techniques.[45,46,48,49] Whereas published clinical guidelines for pre-manipulative assessment for the cervical spine focus upon minimizing risks associated with thrust techniques, it should be noted that these precautions should apply equally to cervical mobilization techniques and cervical traction.[124] Vascular risk assessment has also been recommended for any cervical treatment procedure involving end range rotation.[125]

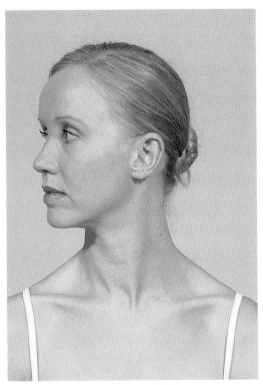

Figure 5.5 Active rotation right.

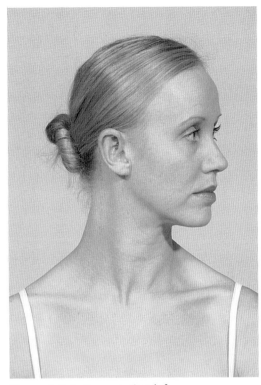

Figure 5.6 Active rotation left.

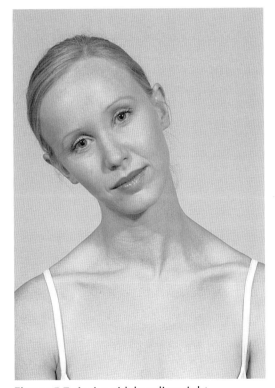

Figure 5.7 Active sidebending right.

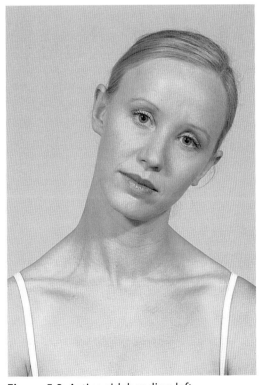

Figure 5.8 Active sidebending left.

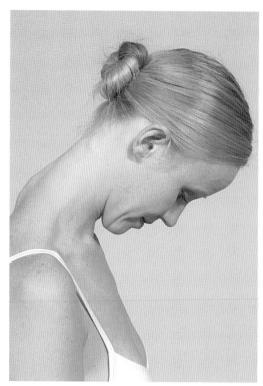

Figure 5.9 Active flexion.

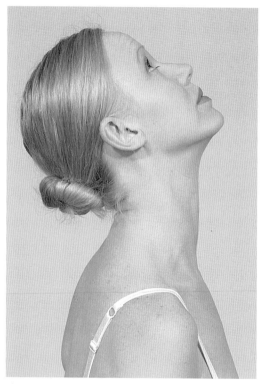

Figure 5.10 Active extension.

Past clinical practice has placed an emphasis on pre-manipulative screening tests to minimize the risk of vertebrobasilar complications as a result of HVLA thrust techniques. It is now recognized that both the vertebral and internal carotid arteries should be considered in pre-treatment risk assessment. Current research would suggest that the emphasis should be placed more on the combination of a thorough patient history, a comprehensive physical examination and the need for a high level of technical skill in the application of HVLA thrust techniques.

UPPER CERVICAL INSTABILITY

The bony anatomy of the atlanto-axial joint favours mobility rather than stability,[126] with the atlanto-axial joint being more vulnerable to subluxation than other segments of the cervical spine.[127] The transverse and alar ligaments have an integral role in maintaining stability in the upper cervical spine. Instability

of the upper cervical spine may compromise related vascular and neurological structures and, in these circumstances, would be a contraindication to the use of HVLA thrust techniques.

Instability must be differentiated from hypermobility.[128,129] Instability is a pathological situation that exists with clinical symptoms or complaints.[128] Causes of upper cervical instability may be a result of incompetence of the odontoid process or the transverse atlantal ligament. These causes can be classified as congenital, inflammatory, neoplastic and traumatic.

Congenital

Incompetence of the odontoid process

- Separate odontoid – 'os odontoideum'
- Free apical segment – 'ossiculum terminale'
- Agenesis of odontoid base
- Agenesis of apical segment
- Agenesis of odontoid process

Incompetence of the transverse atlantal ligament

- Idiopathic
- Down's syndrome

Inflammatory

Incompetence of the odontoid process

- Osteomyelitis

Incompetence of the transverse atlantal ligament

- Bacterial infection
- Viral infection
- Granulomatous change
- Rheumatoid arthritis
- Ankylosing spondylitis

Neoplastic

Incompetence of the odontoid process

- Primary tumour of bone
- Metastatic tumour of bone

Traumatic

Incompetence of the odontoid process

- Acute bony injury
- Chronic bony change

Incompetence of the transverse atlantal ligament

- Acute ligamentous damage associated with fracture and trauma
- Chronic ligamentous change

Symptoms and signs of upper cervical instability

Symptomatic instability of the upper cervical spine is rare. Instability occurs most frequently in patients with rheumatoid arthritis (Fig. 5.11)[130] and is also well documented in Down's syndrome[131–134] and in patients subsequent to retropharyngeal inflammatory processes.[135] Ligamentous laxity following an infectious process in the head or neck occurs most frequently in children, but it is a rare complication. Adult cases have also been

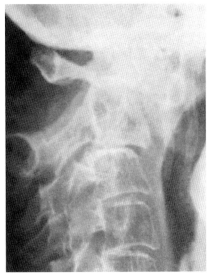

Figure 5.11 Cervical instability as a result of rheumatoid arthritis. Note forward displacement of C1 upon C2 and widening of the atlanto-dental interval.
(Reproduced with permission from Elsevier from Adams and Hamblen, 2001.[130])

reported.[135] Between 7% and 30% of all individuals with Down's syndrome show atlanto-axial instability with most of the patients with radiographic evidence of instability being asymptomatic.[136] Upper cervical ligamentous injuries and instability can also result from trauma.[137,138]

The ability to recognize symptoms and signs that may indicate upper cervical instability is essential for safe practice. These symptoms are extremely variable and might include:[129]

- Neck pain
- Limitation of neck movements
- Torticollis
- Neurological symptoms
- Headache
- Dizziness
- Buzzing in the ears
- Dysphagia
- Neurological signs
- Hyper-reflexia
- Gait disturbances
- Spasticity
- Pareses

The above symptoms and signs might also indicate the presence of cervical artery dysfunction or spinal cord compression unrelated to upper cervical instability. As a result, it is necessary to establish whether the symptoms or signs are related to instability of the upper cervical spine or to other causes.

There are four cardinal symptoms and signs that may indicate the presence of upper cervical instability.[139]

1. Overt loss of balance in relation to head movements.
2. Facial lip paraesthesia, reproduced by active or passive neck movements.
3. Bilateral or quadrilateral limb paraesthesia either constant or reproduced by neck movements.
4. Nystagmus produced by active or passive neck movements.

Currently the most reliable method for detecting increased movement in the upper cervical spine is by the use of imaging techniques. The atlanto-dental interval is the distance between the most anterior point of the dens of the axis and the back of the anterior arch of the atlas. This is measured on lateral radiographs of the cervical spine in flexion, neutral and extension positions. An atlanto-dental interval > 2.5–3 mm in adults and > 4.5–5 mm in children indicates atlanto-axial instability.[136] Cineradiography has also been shown to be a valuable adjunctive technique in the diagnosis of cervical instability.[140] CT may have some advantages over plain radiographs[141] with MRI also offering benefits because of the ability to provide direct sagittal projection.[136]

CT and MRI provide complementary information when combined with flexion and extension radiographs. However, caution should be used when using flexion and extension views in cases of acute cervical trauma.[142]

A number of physical tests have been described for the examination of instability of the upper cervical region.[136,139,143–145] Although these tests are used in clinical practice the results should be interpreted with caution as there is little research evidence confirming their clinical utility.

Tests have been described for both the transverse atlantal and alar ligaments. However, caution must be exercised when interpreting these tests if a practitioner relies solely upon the amount of palpable displacement and end feel.[136] It has been reported that tests of passive intervertebral movement in the upper cervical spine in whiplash-associated disorders corresponded reasonably well with MRI assessment, suggesting potential clinical utility.[146] When screening for upper cervical instability, consideration should also be given to symptom reproduction or modification.

Transverse atlantal ligament stress test

The Sharp–Purser test was designed to demonstrate anterior instability at the atlanto-axial segment in patients with rheumatoid arthritis and ankylosing spondylitis.[143,145] A modified Sharp–Purser test analyses the onset of symptoms and signs following head and neck flexion and the reduction of signs and symptoms accompanying posterior translation of the occiput and atlas on the axis.

Patient position
Sitting with the head and neck relaxed in a semi-flexed position.

Operator position
Standing to the right of the patient with your right arm cradling the patient's forehead. The spinous process and vertebral arch of the axis is stabilized with your thumb and index finger of your left hand (Fig. 5.12).

Stress applied
The occiput and atlas are translated posteriorly by applying pressure on the forehead with your right arm (Fig. 5.13).

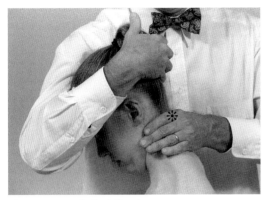

Figure 5.12 ✳ Stabilization.

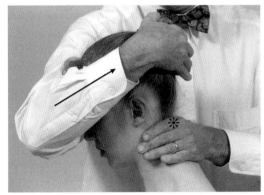

Figure 5.13 ✳ Stabilization. ➔ Plane of force (operator).

Positive test

A positive test occurs with:

1. First onset of symptoms and signs with head and neck flexion.
2. Reduction of symptoms and signs with posterior translation of the occiput and atlas on the axis.
3. Palpable hypermobility of anterior / posterior translation.

Alar ligament stress tests

There are many tests that purport to stress the alar ligaments and identify alar ligament instability. A comprehensive testing regime might include the following three tests.

1. Patient sitting with the neck in a neutral position. Ensure that there is no sidebending of the head and neck. The

operator stabilizes the spinous process and vertebral arch of the axis with thumb and index finger. Passively rotate the occiput and atlas to the right (Fig. 5.14). There should be no more than 20–30° rotation. Repeat the procedure to the left.
A positive test is characterized by the onset of symptoms or signs and / or a range of passive rotation greater than 30° at the upper cervical segments.
2. Patient sitting with the neck in a neutral position. Ensure the head is straight and there is no rotation of the neck. The operator stabilizes the spinous process and vertebral arch of the axis with thumb and index finger while placing the other hand on the patient's vertex (Fig. 5.15). Attempt to passively sidebend the head to the left and then the right (Fig. 5.16). There should be minimal movement in either direction. This test must be repeated with the neck in flexion (Fig. 5.17) and extension (Fig. 5.18).
A positive test is characterized by the onset of symptoms or signs and / or an increased range of passive sidebending in all positions of neutral, flexion and extension.

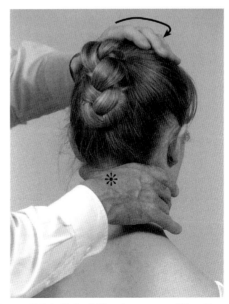

Figure 5.14 ✳ Stabilization. ⟶ Direction of body movement.

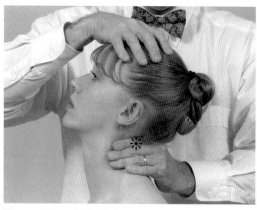

Figure 5.15 ❋ Stabilization.

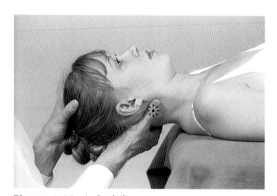

Figure 5.18 ❋ Stabilization.

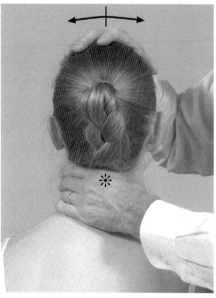

Figure 5.16 ❋ Stabilization. ←→ Direction of body movement.

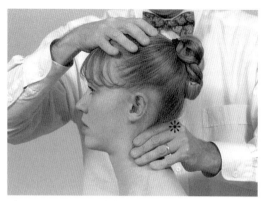

Figure 5.19 ❋ Stabilization

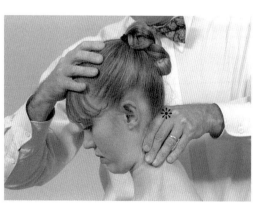

Figure 5.17 ❋ Stabilization.

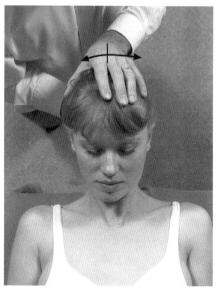

Figure 5.20 ←→ Direction of body movement.

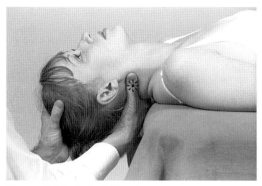

Figure 5.21 ✳ Stabilization.

3. Patient supine with the head and neck beyond the end of the couch and in a neutral position. Ensure the head is straight and there is no rotation of the neck. The operator stabilizes the spinous process and vertebral arch of the axis with thumb and index finger while placing the other hand on the patient's vertex (Fig. 5.19). Both hands support the weight of the patient's head. Attempt to passively sidebend the head to the left and then the right. There should be minimal movement in either direction. This test must be repeated with the neck in flexion (Fig. 5.20) and extension (Fig. 5.21). A positive test is characterized by the onset of symptoms or signs and / or an increased range of passive sidebending in all positions of neutral, flexion and extension.

Transverse atlantal and alar ligament stress tests have been developed on the premise that patients at risk from manipulation to the upper cervical spine may be identified using physical examination techniques. There is a need for continuing research to investigate the reliability and validity of upper cervical instability tests in identifying those patients at risk.

Informed consent

Informed consent may be defined as: 'the voluntary and revocable agreement of a competent individual to participate in a therapeutic or research procedure, based on an adequate understanding of its nature, purpose and implications'.[147] Informed consent comprises four elements, each of which should be present to a satisfactory degree if consent is to be valid (Fig. 5.22).[148]

When a health practitioner provides information to a patient it should be free of any controlling or coercive influences. The information should also be presented in a relevant and meaningful manner that is both intellectually and emotionally comprehensible to the patient.[149]

Information exchange

The traditional method of communication in the clinical encounter is verbal, but this form of communication can be enhanced by written information. To be effective, the written information should be both legible and readable.[150] Videotaped material has also been shown to be effective in patient education particularly with regard to short-term knowledge.[151] Delany[152] advocates that a combination of verbal, written and audiovisual information be provided to patients.

The following have been identified as key elements for obtaining informed consent in clinical practice:[153]

- Discussion of the clinical issue and the nature of the decision to be made
- Discussion of the alternatives
- Discussion of the benefits and risks of alternatives

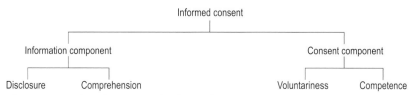

Figure 5.22 The elements of informed consent. (From Sim, 1996.[148])

Box 5.3 Informed consent – practitioner checklist

- Discuss the clinical findings
- Discuss manipulation and why this treatment is recommended
- Demonstrate manipulation treatment using videotaped material
- Discuss alternative treatment approaches
- Discuss the benefits and risks of manipulation and treatment alternatives
- Discuss the uncertainties that arise from the conflicting evidence as to the benefits and risks of manipulation and the treatment alternatives
- Assess the patient's understanding of the information provided
- Discuss the patient's preference for treatment
- Ask the patient to sign a consent form

- Discussion of uncertainties associated with the decision
- Assessment of the patient's understanding
- Asking patients to express their preference.

A suggested checklist prior to applying a HVLA thrust technique is outlined in Box 5.3.

CONCLUSION

It is often stated that manipulation of the spine is a therapeutic technique associated with a high level of risk.

The potential benefits for the patient must be weighed against the risks associated with manipulation of the cervical spine.[154–156] There are currently no high-quality data to enable accurate estimation of the risk of stroke following cervical manipulation or establish causation.[157] Although there is a temporal relationship it may not be a causal relationship. If there is a potential for serious sequelae, the risk appears to be extremely low.[158,159]

The evidence review accompanying the national clinical guidelines on acute and recurrent low back pain indicates that the risks of manipulation for low back pain are very low provided patients are assessed and selected for treatment by trained practitioners.[160,161]

The risk of a serious adverse event following neck manipulation is considered to be low to very low.[162] A review of the literature relating to the risk of neurovascular compromise complicating cervical spine manipulation concluded that an analysis of the risks and benefits supports the continued judicial use of cervical spine manipulation by a prudent and appropriately trained practitioner.[158]

An extensive review of the literature indicates that the key to safety is dependent upon appropriate training, a thorough patient history and physical assessment prior to the application of any manipulative procedure. Appropriate training in the use of manipulative thrust techniques and subsequent skill refinement through regular practice are key elements for safe practice and professional competence.[163]

References

1 Carey P. A report on the occurrence of cerebral vascular accidents in chiropractic practice. J Can Chiropractic Assoc 1993;37:104–106.

2 Dabbs V, Lauretti W. A risk assessment of cervical manipulation vs NSAIDs for the treatment of neck pain. J Manipulative Physiol Ther 1995;18:530–536.

3 Dvorak J, Orelli F. How dangerous is manipulation to the cervical spine? J Man Med 1985;2:1–4.

4 Dvorak J, Loustalot D, Baumgartner H, et al. Frequency of complications of manipulations of the spine. A survey among the members of the Swiss medical society of manual medicine. Eur Spine J 1993;2:136–139.

5 Gutmann G. Injuries to the vertebral artery caused by manual therapy. Man Med 1983;21:2–14.

6 Haldeman S, Kohlbeck F, McGregor M. Unpredictability of cerebrovascular ischemia associated with cervical spine manipulation therapy: a review of sixty four cases after cervical spine manipulation. Spine 2002;27 (1):49–55.

7 Haynes M. Stroke following cervical manipulation in Perth. Chiropractic J Aust 1994;24:42–46.

8 Jaskoviak P. Complications arising from manipulation of the cervical spine. J Manipulative Physiol Ther 1980;3:213–219.

9 Klougart N, Leboeuf-Yde C, Rasmussen LR. Safety in chiropractic practice, Part 1: the occurrence of cerebrovascular accidents after manipulation to the neck in Denmark from 1978–1988. J Manipulative Physiol Ther 1996;19:371–377.

10 Lee KP, Carlini WG, McCormick GF, et al. Neurologic complications following chiropractic manipulation: a survey of California neurologists. Neurology 1995;45:1213–1215.

11 Patijn J. Complications in manual medicine: a review of the literature. J Man Med 1991;6:89–92.

12 Rivett DA, Milburn PA. A prospective study of cervical spine manipulation. J Man Med 1996;4:166–170.

13 Rivett D, Reid D. Risk of stroke for cervical spine manipulation in New Zealand. N Z J Physiother 1998;26:14–17.

14 Miley M, Wellik K, Wingerchuk D, et al. Does cervical manipulative therapy cause vertebral artery dissection and stroke? Neurologist 2008;14 (1):66–73.

15 Coulter ID, Hurwitz EL, Adams AH, et al. The Appropriateness of Manipulation and Mobilization of the Cervical Spine. CA: RAND: Santa Monica; 1996.

16 Reid D, Hing W. AJP Forum: Pre-manipulative testing of the cervical spine. Aust J Physiother 2001;47:164.

17 Powell FC, Hanigan WC, Olivero WC. A risk / benefit analysis of spinal manipulation therapy for relief of lumbar or cervical pain. Neurosurgery 1993;33:73–79.

18 Ernst E. Manipulation of the cervical spine: A systematic review of case reports of serious adverse events, 1995–2001. Med J Aust 2002;176 (8):376–380.

19 Ernst E. Adverse effects of spinal manipulation: A systematic review. J R Soc Med 2007;100 (7):330–338.

20 Di Fabio RP. Manipulation of the cervical spine: Risks and benefits. Phys Ther 1999;79(1):51–65.

21 Haldeman S, Kohlbeck F, McGregor M. Risk factors and precipitating neck movements causing vertebrobasilar artery dissection after cervical trauma and spinal manipulation. Spine 1999;24(8):785–794.

22 Endo K, Ichimaru K, Shimura H, Imakiire A. Cervical vertigo after hair shampoo treatment at a hairdressing salon: a case report. Spine 2000;25 (5):632–634.

23 Haneline M, Lewkovich G. An analysis of the etiology of cervical artery dissections: 1994 to 2003. J Manipulative Physiol Ther 2005;28 (8):617–622.

24 Taylor A, Kerry R. Neck pain and headache as a result of internal carotid artery dissection: implications for manual therapists. Man Ther 2005;10(1):73–77.

25 Rubinstein S, Haldeman S, van-Tulder M. An etiologic model to help explain the pathogenesis of cervical artery dissection: Implications for cervical manipulation. J Manipulative Physiol Ther 2006;29(4):336–338.

26 Maroon J, Gardner P, Abla A, et al. Golfer's stroke: Golf-induced stroke from vertebral artery dissection. Surg Neurol 2007;67(2):163–168.

27 Schneck M, Simionescu M, Bijari A. Bilateral vertebral artery dissection possibly precipitated in delayed fashion as a result of roller coaster rides. Journal of Stroke and Cerebrovascular diseases 2008;17(1):39–41.

28 Cassidy J, Boyle E, Cote P, et al. Risk of Vertebrobasilar stroke and chiropractic care. Results of a population-based case-control and case-crossover study. Spine 2008;33 (4S):176–183.

29 Smith W, Johnston S, Skalabrin E, et al. Spinal manipulative therapy is an independent risk factor for vertebral artery dissection. Neurology 2003;60(9):1424–1428.

30 Williams L, Biller J. Vertebrobasilar dissection and cervical spine manipulation: A complex pain in the neck. Neurology 2003;60(9):1408–1409.

31 Haldeman S, Carey P, Townsend M, et al. Clinical perceptions of the risk of vertebral artery dissection after cervical manipulation: The effect of referral bias. Spine J 2002;2(5):334–342.

32 Oppenheim J, Spitzer D, Segal D. Nonvascular complications following spinal manipulation. Spine J 2005;5(6):660–667.

33 Chou R, Huffman L. Non pharmacologic therapies for acute and chronic low back pain: A review of the evidence for an American Pain Society / American College of Physicians clinical practice guideline. Ann Intern Med 2007;147 (7):492–504.

34 Meeker W, Haldeman S. Chiropractic: A profession at the crossroads of mainstream and alternative medicine. Ann Intern Med 2002;136 (3):216–227.

35 Oliphant D. Safety of spinal manipulation in the treatment of lumbar disk herniations: A systematic review and risk assessment. J Manipulative Physiol Ther 2004;27(3):197–210.

36 Haldeman S. Authors reply to Dr Oppenheim et al. Nonvascular complications following spinal manipulation. Spine J 2006;6(4):474–475.

37 Thiel H, Bolton J, Docherty S, et al. Safety of chiropractic manipulation of the cervical spine. A prospective national survey. Spine 2007;32 (21):2375–2378.

38 Hurwitz E, Morgenstern H, Vassilaki M, et al. Frequency and clinical predictors of adverse reactions to chiropractic care in the UCLA neck pain study. Spine 2005;30(13):1477–1484.

39 Senstad O, Leboeuf-Yde C, Borchgrevink C. Frequency and characteristics of side effects of spinal manipulative therapy. Spine 1997;22 (4):435–440.

40 Leboeuf-Yde C, Hennius B, Rudberg E, et al. Side effects of chiropractic treatment: A prospective study. J Manipulative Physiol Ther 1997;20 (8):511–515.

41 Cagnie B, Vinck E, Beernaert A, et al. How common are side effects of spinal manipulation and can these side effects be predicted? Man Ther 2004;9(3):151–156.

42 Rubinstein S, Leboeuf-Yde C, Knol D, et al. The benefits outweigh the risks for patients undergoing chiropractic care for neck pain: A prospective, multicenter, cohort study. J Manipulative Physiol Ther 2007;30(6):408–418.

43 Rubinstein S, Leboeuf-Yde C, Knol D, et al. Predictors of adverse events following chiropractic care for patient's with neck pain. J Manipulative Physiol Ther 2008;31(2):93–103.

44 Donovan J, Kerber C, Donovan W, et al. Development of spontaneous intracranial hypotension concurrent with grade IV mobilization of the cervical and thoracic spine: A case report. Arch Phys Med Rehabil 2007;88 (11):1472–1473.

45 Michaeli A. Reported occurrence and nature of complications following manipulative physiotherapy in South Africa. Aust Physiotherapy 1993;39(4):309–315.

46 Jumper J, Horton J. Central retinal artery occlusion after manipulation of the neck by a chiropractor. Am J Opthalmol 1996;121 (3):321–322.

47 Tsuboi K. Retinal and cerebral artery embolism after 'shiatsu' on the neck. Stroke 2001;32 (10):2441.

48 Grant A, Wang N. Carotid dissection associated with a handheld electric massager. Southern Med J 2004;97(12):1262–1263.

49 Magarey M, Rebbeck T, Coughlan B, et al. Pre-manipulative testing of the cervical spine: review, revision and new clinical guidelines. Man Ther 2004;9(2):95–108.

50 Dabbs V, Lauretti W. A risk assessment of cervical manipulation vs. NSAIDs for the treatment of neck pain. J Manipulative Physiol Ther 1995;18 (8):530–536.

51 Vincent C. The safety of acupuncture. BMJ 2001;323(7311):467–468.

52 Rivett D, Shirley D, Magarey M, et al. Clinical Guidelines for Assessing Vertebrobasilar Insufficiency in the Management of Cervical Spine Disorders. Melbourne, Victoria: Australian Physiotherapy Association; 2006.

53 Annual Report 2008. International Air Transport Association (IATA):22. http://www.iata.org/index.htm.

54 Sizer P, Brismee J, Cook C. Medical screening for red flags in the diagnosis and management of musculoskeletal spine pain. Pain Pract 2007;7 (1):53–71.

55 Edelman RR, Hesselink JD, Zlatkin MB, Crues JV. Clinical Magnetic Resonance Imaging, 3rd Edn. Philadelphia: Saunders; 2009.

56 Boden S, Davis D, Dina T, et al. Abnormal magnetic-resonance scans of the lumbar spine in asymptomatic subjects. J Bone & Joint Surg Am 1990;72-A(3):403–408.

57 Jensen M, Brant-Zawadzki M, Obuchowski N, et al. Magnetic resonance imaging of the lumbar spine in people without back pain. N Engl J Med 1994;331(2):69–73.

58 Boos N, Rieder R, Schade V, et al. The diagnostic accuracy of magnetic resonance imaging, work perception, and psychosocial factors in identifying symptomatic disc herniations. Spine 1995;20(4):2613–2625.

59 Brant-Zawadzki M, Jensen M, Obuchowski N, et al. Interobserver and intraobserver variability in interpretation of lumbar disc abnormalities. Spine 1995;20(11):1257–1264.

60 Wood K, Blair J, Aepple D, et al. The natural history of asymptomatic thoracic disc herniations. Spine 1997;22(5):525–529.

61 Borenstein D, O'Mara J, Boden S, et al. The value of magnetic resonance imaging of the lumbar spine to predict low-back pain in asymptomatic subjects. J Bone & Joint Surg Am 2001;83-A(9):1306–1311.

62 Ernst C, Stadnik T, Peeters E, et al. Prevalence of annular tears and disc herniations on MR images of the cervical spine in symptom free volunteers. Eur J Radiol 2005;55(3): 409–414.

63 Santillia V, Beghi E, Finucci S. Chiropractic manipulation in the treatment of acute back pain and sciatica with disc protrusion: A randomized double-blind clinical trial of active and simulated spinal manipulations. Spine J 2006;6 (2):131–137.

64 Cyriax R. Textbook of Orthopaedic Medicine1984;Vol 2:London: Baillière Tindall; 1984.

65 Maigne R. Diagnosis and Treatment of Pain of Vertebral Origin: A Manual Medicine Approach. Baltimore, MD: Williams & Wilkins; 1996.

66 BenEliyahu D. Magnetic resonance imaging and clinical follow-up: Study of 27 patients receiving chiropractic care for cervical and lumbar disc herniations. J Manipulative Physiol Ther 1996;19 (9):597–606.

67 Herzog W. Clinical Biomechanics of Spinal Manipulation. New York, NY: Churchill Livingstone; 2000.

68 Burton A, Tillotson K, Cleary J. Single-blind randomised controlled trial of chemonucleolysis and manipulation in the treatment of symptomatic lumbar disc herniation. Eur Spine J 2000;9(3):202–207.

69 McMorland G, Suter E, Casha S, et al. Manipulation or microdiscectomy for sciatica: A prospective randomized controlled trial. Spine J 2007;7(5):1S–66S.

70 Snelling N. Spinal manipulation in patients with disc herniation: A critical review of risk and benefit. Int J Osteopath Med 2006;9 (3):77–84.

71 Tseng S, Lin S, Chen Y, et al. Ruptured cervical disc after spinal manipulation therapy. Spine 2002;27(3):E80–E82.

72 Haldeman S, Rubinstein S. Cauda equina syndrome in patients undergoing manipulation of the lumbar spine. Spine 1992;17(12):1469–1473.

73 Markowitz H, Dolce D. Cauda equina syndrome due to sequestrated recurrent disk herniation after chiropractic manipulation. Orthopedics 1997;20 (7):652–653.

74 Lisi A, Holmes E, Ammendolia C. High-velocity low-amplitude spinal manipulation for symptomatic lumbar disk disease: A systematic review of the literature. J Manipulative Physiol Ther 2005;28(6):429–442.

75 CSAG. Back pain. Clinical Standards Advisory Group Report. London: HMSO; 1994.

76 Rubinstein S, Peerdeman S, van Tulder M, et al. A systematic review of the risk factors for cervical artery dissection. Stroke 2005;36(7): 1575–1580.

77 Dittrich R, Rohsbach D, Heidbreder A, et al. Mild mechanical traumas are possible risk factors for cervical artery dissection. Cerebrovasc Dis 2007;23(4):275–281.

78 Arnold M, Cumurciuc R, Stapf C, et al. Pain as the only symptom of cervical artery dissection. J Neurol Neurosurg Psychiatry 2006;77 (9):1021–1024.

79 Shibata T, Kubo M, Kuwayama N, et al. Warning headache of subarachnoid hemorrhage and infarction due to vertebrobasilar artery dissection. Clin J Pain 2006;22(2):193–196.

80 Lumley J. Surface Anatomy, 2nd edn. New York, NY: Churchill Livingstone; 1996: 23.

81 Zweibel WJ. Introduction to Vascular Ultrasonography, 2nd edn. New York, NY: Harcourt Brace; 1986.

82 Rivett D. The premanipulative vertebral artery testing protocol. N Z J Physiother 1995(April): 9-12.

83 Silbert P, Mokri B, Schievink W. Headache and neck pain in spontaneous internal carotid and vertebral artery dissections. Neurology 1995;45:1517–1522.

84 Schievink W. Spontaneous dissection of the carotid and vertebral arteries. N Engl J Med 2001;344:898–906.

85 Barker S, Kesson M, Ashmore J, et al. Guidance for pre-manipulative testing of the cervical spine. Man Ther 2000;5(1):37–40.

86 Maigne R. Orthopaedic Medicine: A New Approach to Vertebral Manipulation. Springfield, IL: Charles C Thomas; 1972.

87 Maitland G. Vertebral Manipulation, 3rd edn. London: Butterworth; 1973.

88 Oostendorp R. Vertebrobasilar insufficiency. Proceedings of the International Federation of Orthopaedic Manipulative Therapists Congress. Cambridge.

89 Terret A. Vascular accidents from cervical spine manipulation: The mechanisms. Australian Chiropractors Association. J Chiropractic 1988;22(5):59–74.

90 Grant R. Vertebral artery insufficiency: A clinical protocol for pre-manipulative testing of the cervical spine. In: Boyling J, Palastanga N eds. Grieve's Modern Manual Therapy, 2nd edn. Edinburgh, UK: Churchill Livingstone; 1994:371–380.

91 Chapman-Smith D. Cervical Adjustment. Chiropractic Rep 1999;13(4):1–7.

92 Brown B, Taltlow W. Radiographic studies of the vertebral arteries in cadavers. Radiology 1963;81:80–88.

93 Toole J, Tucker S. Influence of head position on cervical circulation. Studies on blood flow in cadavers. Arch Neurol 1960;2: 616–623.

94 Refshauge K. Rotation: a valid premanipulative dizziness test? Does it predict safe manipulation? J Manipulative Physiol Ther 1994;17(1):15–19.

95 Rivett D, Sharples K, Milburn PD. Effect of pre-manipulative test on vertebral artery and internal carotid artery blood flow: a pilot study. J Manipulative Physiol Ther 1999;22:368–375.

96 Zaina C, Grant R, Johnson C, et al. The effect of cervical rotation on blood flow in the

contralateral vertebral artery. Man Ther 2003;8 (2):103–109.

97 Arnold C, Bourassa R, Langer T, et al. Doppler studies evaluating the effect of a physical therapy screening protocol on vertebral artery blood flow. Man Ther 2004;9(1):13–21.

98 Tissington-Tatlow W, Bammer H. Syndrome of vertebral artery compression. Neurology 1957;7:331–340.

99 Toole J, Tucker S. Influence of head position on cerebral circulation. Arch Neurol 1960;2:616–623.

100 Schmitt H. Anatomical structure of the cervical spine with reference to pathology of manipulation complications. J Man Med 1991;6:93–101.

101 Stevens A. Functional Doppler sonography of the vertebral artery and some considerations about manual techniques. J Man Med 1991;6:102–105.

102 Haynes M. Doppler studies comparing the effects of cervical rotation and lateral flexion on vertebral artery blood flow. J Manipulative Physiol Ther 1996;19:378–384.

103 Mitchell J. Changes in vertebral artery blood flow following normal rotation of the cervical spine. J Manipulative Physiol Ther 2003;26(6):347–351.

104 Mitchell J, Keene D, Dyson C, et al. Is cervical spine rotation, as used in the standard vertebrobasilar insufficiency test, associated with a measurable change in intracranial vertebral artery blood flow? Man Ther 2004;9(4):220–227.

105 Licht P, Christensen H, Hojgaard P, et al. Triplex ultrasound of vertebral artery flow during cervical rotation. J Manipulative Physiol Ther 1998;21:27–31.

106 Licht P, Christensen H, Hoilund-Carlsen P. Vertebral artery volume flow in human beings. J Manipulative Physiol Ther 1999;22:363–367.

107 Licht P, Christensen H, Hoilund-Carlsen P. Is there a role for pre-manipulative testing before cervical manipulation. J Manipulative Physiol Ther 2000;23:175–179.

108 Haynes M, Milne N. Color duplex sonographic findings in human vertebral arteries during cervical rotation. J Clin Ultrasound 2000;29:14–24.

109 Haynes M, Cala L, Melsom A, et al. Vertebral arteries and cervical rotation: Modeling and magnetic resonance angiography studies. J Manipulative Physiol Ther 2002;25(6):370–383.

110 Gross A, Chesworth B, Binkley J. A case for evidence based practice in manual therapy. In: Boyling J, Jull G eds. Grieve's Modern Manual Therapy – The Vertebral Column, 3rd edn. Edinburgh, UK: Churchill Livingstone; 2005: Ch. 39.

111 Richter R, Reinking M. Evidence in practice. How does evidence on the diagnostic accuracy of the vertebral artery test influence teaching of the test in a professional physical therapist education program? Phys Ther 2005;85 (6):589–599.

112 Thiel H, Wallace K, Donat J, et al. Effect of various head and neck positions on vertebral artery flow. Clin Biomechanics 1994;9:105–110.

113 Cote P, Kreitz B, Cassidy J, et al. The validity of the extension–rotation test as a clinical screening procedure before neck manipulation: A secondary analysis. J Manipulative Physiol Ther 1996;19(3):159–164.

114 Rivett D, Milburn P, Chapple C. Negative pre-manipulative vertebral artery testing despite complete occlusion: a case of false negativity. Man Ther 1998;3(2):102–107.

115 Licht P, Christensen H, Hoilund-Carlsen P. Carotid artery blood flow during premanipulative testing. J Manipulative Physiol Ther 2002;25(9):568–572.

116 Westaway M, Stratford P, Symons B. False-negative extension / rotation pre-manipulative screening test on a patient with an atretic and hypoplastic vertebral artery. Man Ther 2003;8 (2):120–127.

117 Grant R. Vertebral artery testing – the Australian Physiotherapy Association Protocol after 6 years. Man Ther 1996;1(3):149–153.

118 Symons B, Leonard T, Herzog W. Internal forces sustained by the vertebral artery during spinal manipulative therapy. J Manipulative Physiol Ther 2002;25(8):504–510.

119 McDermaid C. Vertebrobasilar incidents and spinal manipulative therapy of the cervical spine. In: Vernon H ed. The Cranio-Cervical Syndrome. Oxford: Butterworth-Heinemann; 2002: Ch. 14.

120 Terrett A. Did the SMT practitioner cause the arterial injury? Chiropractic J Aust 2002;32 (3):99–119.

121 Thiel H, Rix G. Is it time to stop functional pre-manipulation testing of the cervical spine? Man Ther 2005;10(2):154–158.

122 Kerry R, Taylor A, Mitchell J, et al. Cervical arterial dysfunction and manual therapy: A critical literature review to inform professional practice. Man Ther 2008;13(4):278–288.

123 Chief Coroner. Inquest Touching the Death of Lana Dale Lewis. Jury Verdict and Recommendations. Province of Ontario, Canada: Office of the Chief Coroner; 2004.

124 Schneider G. Vertebral artery complications following gentle cervical treatments. Aust J Physiother 2002;48(2):151.

125 Australian Physiotherapy Association (APA). Clinical Guidelines for assessing vertebrobasilar

insufficiency in the management of cervical spine disorders. Online. Available: www. physiotherapy.asn.au; 2006.

126 Penning L, Wilmink J. Rotation of the cervical spine, a CT study in normals. Spine 1987;12 (8):732–738.

127 Louri H, Stewart W. Spontaneous atlantoaxial dislocation. N Engl J Med 1961;265(14):677–681.

128 Swinkels R, Beeton K, Alltree J. Pathogenesis of upper cervical instability. Man Ther 1996;1 (3):127–132.

129 Swinkels R, Oostendorp R. Upper cervical instability: fact or fiction. J Manipulative Physiol Ther 1996;19(3):185–194.

130 Adams JC, Hamblen DL. Outline of Orthopaedics. Edinburgh, UK: Churchill Livingstone; 2001: Ch. 9.

131 Tredwell S, Newman D, Lockitch G. Instability of the upper cervical spine in Down syndrome. J Pediatr Orthop 1990;10:602–606.

132 Gabriel K, Mason D, Carango P. Occipito-atlantal translation in Down's syndrome. Spine 1990;15:997–1002.

133 Parfenchuck T, Bertrand S, Powers M, et al. Posterior occipitoatlantal hypermobility in Down syndrome: An analysis of 199 patients. J Pediatr Orthop 1994;14:304–308.

134 Matsuda Y, Sano N, Watanabe S, et al. Atlanto-occipital hypermobility in subjects with Down's syndrome. Spine 1995;20 (21):2283–2286.

135 Ugur H, Caglar S, Unlu A, et al. Infection-related atlantoaxial subluxation in two adults: Grisel syndrome or not? Acta Neurochir 2003;145:69–72.

136 Cattrysse E, Swinkels R, Oostendorp R, et al. Upper cervical instability: are clinical tests reliable? Man Ther 1997;2(2):91–97.

137 Chiu W, Haan J, Cushing B, et al. Ligamentous injuries of the cervical spine in unreliable blunt trauma patients: Incidence, evaluation and outcome.. J Trauma Inj, Infection, and Critical Care 2001;50(3):457–464.

138 Dickman C, Greene K, Sonntag V. Injuries involving the transverse atlantal ligament: Classification and treatment guidelines based upon experience with 39 injuries. Neurosurgery 1996;38(1):44–50.

139 Pettman E. Stress tests of the craniovertebral joints. In: Boyling J, Palastanga N eds. Grieve's Modern Manual Therapy. Edinburgh, UK: Churchill Livingstone; 1994: Ch. 38.

140 Hino H, Abumi K, Kanayama M, et al. Dynamic motion analysis of normal and unstable cervical spines using cineradiography. Spine 1999;24 (2):163–168.

141 Roach J, Duncan D, Wenger D, et al. Atlanto-axial instability and spinal cord compression in children – diagnosis by computerized tomography. J Bone Jt Surg (Am Vol) 1984;66:708–714.

142 Dickman C, Greene K, Sonntag V. Injuries involving the transverse atlantal ligament: Classification and treatment guidelines based upon experience with 39 injuries. Neurosurgery 1996;38(1):44–50.

143 Sharp J, Purser D. Spontaneous atlantoaxial dislocation in ankylosing spondylitis and rheumatoid arthritis. Ann Rheum Dis 1961;20:47–77.

144 Uitvlught G, Indenbaum S. Clinical assessment of atlantoaxial instability using the Sharp–Purser test. Arthritis Rheum 1988;31(7):370–374.

145 Meadows J. The Sharp–Purser Test: A useful clinical tool or an exercise in futility and risk? J Man Manipulative Ther 1998;6(2):97–100.

146 Kaale B, Krakenes J, Albrektsen G, et al. Clinical assessment techniques for detecting ligament and membrane injuries in the upper cervical spine region – a comparison with MRI results. Man Ther 2008;13(5):397–403.

147 Sim J. Informed consent: Ethical implications for physiotherapy. Physiotherapy 1986;72:584.

148 Sim J. Informed consent and manual therapy. Man Ther 1996;2:104–106.

149 Delany C. Informed consent: Broadening the focus. Aust J Physiother 2003;49:159–161.

150 Albert T, Chadwick S. How readable are practice leaflets. BMJ 1992;305(6864):1266–1268.

151 Gagliano M. A literature review on the efficacy of video in patient education. J Med Educ 1988;63 (10):785–792.

152 Delany C. Cervical manipulation – How might informed consent be obtained before treatment? J Law Med 2002;10(2):174–186.

153 Braddock C, Fihn S, Levinson W, et al. How doctors and patients discuss routine clinical decisions. Informed decision making in the out-patient setting. J Gen Intern Med 1997;12 (6):339–345.

154 Spitzer W, Skovron M, Salmi L, et al. Monograph of the Quebec task force on whiplash-associated disorders: redefining whiplash and its management. Spine 1995;20:8S.

155 Hurwitz E, Aker P, Adams A, et al. Manipulation and mobilization of the cervical spine: A systematic review of the literature. Spine 1996;21 (15):1746–1760.

156 Miley M, Wellik K, Wingerchuk D, et al. Does cervical manipulative therapy cause vertebral artery dissection and stroke? The Neurologist 2008;14(1):66–73.

157 Breen A. Manipulation of the neck and stroke: time for more rigorous evidence. Med J Aust 2002;176:364–365.

158 Rivett D. Neurovascular compromise complicating cervical spine manipulation: What is the risk? J Man Manipulative Ther 1995;3 (4):144–151.

159 Clubb D. Cervical manipulation and vertebral artery injury: A literature review. J Man Manipulative Ther 2002;10(1):11–16.

160 Royal College of General Practitioners. Clinical Guidelines on Acute and Recurrent Low Back Pain. London: Royal College of General Practitioners; 1996:Ch. 2.

161 Waddell G. The Back Pain Revolution. Edinburgh, UK: Churchill Livingstone; 1998: Ch. 16.

162 Thiel H, Bolton J, Docherty S, et al. Safety of chiropractic manipulation of the cervical spine: A prospective national survey. Spine 2007;32 (21):2375–2378.

163 Vick D, McKay C, Zengerle C. The safety of manipulative treatment: Review of the literature from 1925 to 1993. J Am Osteopath Assoc 1996;96(2):113–115.

6

Rationale for the use of HVLA thrust techniques

High-velocity low-amplitude (HVLA) thrust techniques are widely used in patient care with increasing evidence of their effectiveness. However, the use of HVLA thrust techniques must be considered within the context of a comprehensive patient management plan, which may include the application of other osteopathic manipulative techniques and adjunctive therapies.

Various authors have described specific indications for the use of HVLA thrust techniques (Box 6.1).

Box 6.1 Specific indications for HVLA thrust techniques as listed by various authors

- Hypomobility[1,2]
- Motion restriction[3–5]
- Joint fixation[6,7]
- Acute joint locking[2,8,9]
- Motion loss with somatic dysfunction[10,11]
- Somatic dysfunction[12–14]
- Restore bony alignment[4,15]
- Meniscoid entrapment[1,3,4,7,16]
- Adhesions[17]
- Displaced disc fragment[18]
- Pain modulation[1,5,9,19,20]
- Reflex relaxation of muscles[1,5,21–23]
- Reprogramming of the central nervous system[12]
- Release of endorphins[24]
- Clinical prediction rule[25–28]

CAVITATION ASSOCIATED WITH HVLA THRUST TECHNIQUES

The aim of HVLA thrust techniques is to achieve joint cavitation that is accompanied by a 'popping' or 'cracking' sound. This audible release distinguishes HVLA procedures from other osteopathic manipulative techniques.

Research involving the metacarpophalangeal joint indicates that the audible release is generated by a cavitation mechanism resulting from a drop in the internal joint pressure.[29–32] Following cavitation, there is an increase in the size of the joint space and gas is found within that space.[29–33] The gas bubble has been described as 80% carbon dioxide[30] or having the density of nitrogen.[14] The gas bubble remains within the joint for between 15 and 30 minutes,[14,29–31,33] which is consistent with the time taken for the gas to be reabsorbed into the synovial fluid.[30] An increased range of joint motion immediately following cavitation has been demonstrated.[33]

The audible release in the lumbar spine is believed to originate from the apophysial joints.[34] Widening of lumbar zygapophysial joints post manipulation has been demonstrated by magnetic resonance imaging (MRI) following lumbar spine manipulation.[35] The situation in the cervical spine is less clear as neck manipulation did not demonstrate similar post-manipulation apophysial joint space widening when assessed using computerized tomography (CT).[36]

A number of studies have reported that thrust techniques are associated with a temporary increase in the range of spinal motion.[37–45] Longer-term effects of HVLA thrust techniques have also been reported[46,47] and it is postulated that these may be due to reflex mechanisms that either directly cause muscle relaxation or inhibit pain.[5] However, the sound of a 'crack' or 'pop' associated with a HVLA thrust technique does not necessarily indicate that reflex or tissue changes have occurred. Some authors have reported benefits from HVLA thrust techniques without the accompanying audible release.[48,49] There continues to be speculation as to the level and side of apophysial joint cavitation when HVLA thrust techniques are applied to the spine.[50–53] It is likely that the level and side of cavitation will be dependent upon a range of factors that might include spinal positioning and locking, the specific technique applied, operator skill and patient compliance and whether the patient is symptomatic or asymptomatic. The aim of HVLA thrust techniques is to achieve cavitation within the normal range of zygapophysial joint motion and not at the anatomical end range.

Repeated 'cracking' or 'popping' of the joints of the hand, associated with cavitation, has not been shown to be linked with an increased incidence of degenerative change.[54,55]

EVIDENCE SUMMARY

Best practice requires practitioners to embrace the principles of evidence-based medicine (EBM). Evidence-based medicine incorporates the best results from clinical and epidemiological research with individual clinical experience and expertise whilst taking account of patient preferences.[56,57]

In manual medicine the focus of critical review of the efficacy of treatment can often be based solely upon research evidence. However clinical experience and patient preferences should also play an important role in deciding the best treatment approach. Practice-based evidence (PBE) is evidence that individual clinicians acquire through clinical experience and practice, which should be informed by research. Best practice should also take account of convention, clinical experience, and patient preference (Fig. 6.1).

Evidence for efficacy of interventions, such as spinal manipulation, can be assessed according to a hierarchy of evidence that exists in the literature for that intervention.

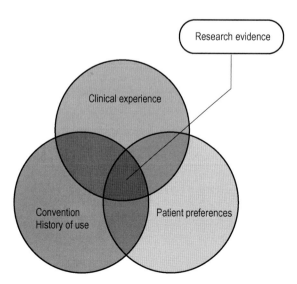

Figure 6.1 Evidence-based medicine.

Hierarchy of evidence

- Randomized controlled trials (RCTs)
- Non-randomized controlled trials
- Cohort or longitudinal studies
- Case-control studies
- Cross-sectional descriptions and surveys
- Case series and case reports
- Expert opinion

Recommendations arising from a review of the research reflect the strength of evidence and methodological quality, but not necessarily the clinical importance.

Research evidence can be synthesized in a number of different ways. A systematic review can be undertaken which is the systematic synthesis of evidence across all trials for a given intervention.

Syntheses

- Systematic reviews including meta-analyses
- Decision and economic analyses
- Guidelines

Meta-analysis is when a systematic review uses special statistical methods for combining the results of several studies. Recommendations based on research evidence can be used to develop clinical practice guidelines and standards for third-party payers and policy makers.

Bronfort et al[58] report that since 1979 there have been in excess of 50 mostly qualitative, non-systematic reviews published relating to manipulation and mobilization treatment for back and neck pain. A number of systematic reviews and meta-analyses have also been undertaken that attempt to determine the efficacy of spinal manipulation on low back pain,[59–69] back and neck pain,[70,71] neck pain[72–76] and chronic headache.[77]

Bronfort et al[71] undertook an extensive search of computerized and bibliographic literature databases up to the end of 2002 relating to the efficacy of spinal manipulation and mobilization for low back and neck pain and concluded that the use of spinal manipulative therapy and / or mobilization is a viable option for the treatment of both low back pain and neck pain. This systematic review identified the paucity of high-quality trials distinguishing between acute and chronic presentations and recommended that further research should examine the value of spinal manipulation and mobilization for well-defined sub-groups of patients and determine the cost-effectiveness of different treatment approaches.

A Cochrane database systematic review on spinal manipulative therapy for low back pain concluded that there is no evidence that spinal manipulation is superior to other standard treatments for patients suffering acute or chronic low back pain.[67] A systematic review of RCTs published since 1995, relating to a range of complementary therapies for non-specific back pain, concluded that spinal manipulation has real but modest benefits for acute and chronic low back pain and that the risks of lumbar manipulation are low.[64] A systematic review relating to chronic low back pain concluded that both spinal manipulation and mobilization are viable treatment options and are at least as effective as other commonly used interventions with a low risk of serious adverse events.[69] Waddell, on reviewing the evidence in relation to acute low back pain and disability, commented that there are numerous symptomatic treatment options other than manipulation but there is little scientific evidence that they are effective and states that the evidence supports the use of manipulation as a treatment option for symptomatic relief.[78] The United Kingdom Back Pain Exercise and Manipulation (UK BEAM) randomized trial concluded that spinal manipulation over a 12-week period produced statistically significant benefits relative to best care in general practice at both 3 and 12 months[79] and that spinal manipulation was also a cost-effective addition to general practice best care.[80] The joint clinical practice guideline from the American College of Physicians and the American Pain Society states that practitioners should consider using spinal manipulation for acute, sub-acute or chronic low back pain in those patients who do not improve with self care options.[81]

A Cochrane review of manipulation and mobilization for mechanical neck pain concluded that, when combined with exercise, mobilization and / or manipulation is beneficial for persistent mechanical neck disorders with or without headache, providing strong evidence for using a multi-modal treatment approach.[74] Vernon et al[75] carried out a systematic analysis of group change scores in RCTs of patients treated with manual therapy suffering from chronic neck pain not due to whiplash and excluding headache or arm pain. They concluded that patients randomized to receive spinal manipulation or mobilization showed clinically important improvements at 6, 12 and up to 104 weeks after treatment. The Bone and Joint Decade 2000–2010 task force on neck pain and its associated disorders reported that the evidence favours supervised exercise sessions with or without manual therapy over usual or no care for both whiplash-associated disorders and neck disorders without trauma.[76] The task force reported that manipulation and mobilization yielded comparable clinical outcomes.

A systematic review of the efficacy of spinal manipulation for chronic headache concluded that spinal manipulative therapy has an effect comparable to commonly prescribed prophylactic tension headache and migraine medications.[77]

In an effort to increase consistency in the management of spinal disorders the available evidence has been reviewed by expert committees to establish clinical guidelines. Clinical guidelines for the management of low back pain have been developed in at least 12 different countries. Since the available evidence is international there would be an expectation that all the guidelines regarding diagnosis and treatment would offer broadly similar recommendations.[81] Willem et al[66] noted that all national guidelines on the management of low back pain included the use of spinal manipulation. However, the data upon which national recommendations are based has been interpreted differently, leading to conflicting guidelines between countries for the use of spinal manipulation in the management of both acute and chronic back pain.

Manual therapy approaches, including HVLA thrust techniques, have been negatively impacted by poorly designed and implemented research studies. Practitioners of manipulative therapy are not a homogeneous group and have differing levels of training and skill in the application of manipulative techniques. Patients with spinal pain are also not a homogeneous group, which makes comparison of like with like extremely difficult. However, practitioners have demonstrated an ability, using signs and symptoms, to identify sub-groups of patients with low back pain and then match them to specific treatment approaches. Those patients matched by the practitioner to specific interventions showed statistically significant improvement compared with non-matched controls.[82] Several classification systems for spinal and pelvic girdle pain have been proposed in an attempt to address this problem and identify the sub-groups of patients who are likely to respond positively to specific interventions.[83–90]

Research into the predictive value of specific clinical findings to identify patients with spinal pain who are likely to benefit from spinal manipulation has led to the development of clinical prediction rules. Clinical prediction rules consist of combinations of variables obtained from self-report measures, patient history and examination that assist in identifying those patients with spinal pain most likely to respond to spinal manipulation.[25–28]

CLINICAL DECISION MAKING

Clinical decision making is the ability to collate and synthesize information, make decisions and appropriately implement these decisions in the clinical environment. At our present state of knowledge, what should guide our clinical decision making to incorporate HVLA thrust techniques within a treatment regimen? All healthcare practitioners utilize a clinical decision-

Box 6.2 Clinical decision making

- Exclude contraindications (red flags)
- Determine influence of yellow flags
- Identify presence of a treatable lesion –
  somatic dysfunction
- Undertake risk–benefit analysis
- Determine patient preferences
- Decide upon appropriate intervention

making process prior to the application of a therapeutic intervention, such as HVLA thrust technique (Box 6.2).

If a patient fails to respond to spinal manipulation the practitioner must reflect upon a number of potential reasons why this might be the case (Box 6.3). Failure of a patient to respond positively may not be a failure due to the technique per se but can result from factors such as initial incorrect choice of technique, inadequate training and poor technical delivery of the technique, inappropriate patient positioning, patient inability to relax and unidentified psychosocial and chronic pain risk factors.

Box 6.3 Failure of therapy

- Therapy effective / ineffective?
- Therapist efficient / inefficient?
- Unidentified psychosocial risk factors?
- Clinical decision making – right / wrong?

Exclude contraindications (red flags)

Although the majority of patients who present with spinal pain will not have serious pathology, it is imperative that practitioners maintain vigilance in excluding red flag conditions (see Contraindications, page 37). The following may indicate the presence of red flags:

- Patient younger than 20 or older than 50 years with first onset of spinal pain
- Pain following trauma
- Constant and worsening pain

- Past or present history of malignancy
- Long-term corticosteroid use
- General malaise
- Night sweats / pyrexia
- Weight loss
- Neurological symptoms and signs

The identification of red flags requires further investigation and specialist referral.

Determine influence of yellow flags

Yellow flags are psychosocial risk factors associated with chronic pain, disability and failure to return to work.[91–99] They are subjective and include negative coping strategies, fear avoidance behaviour, anxiety, depression and distress. Practitioners should screen for yellow flags (adverse prognostic factors) and, if identified, treatment should aim to reduce dependency on medication and other passive forms of treatment, including manipulative therapy, and encourage the development of self-management skills. Despite widespread study, uncertainty remains regarding which risk factors for poor recovery are associated with particular outcomes and the strength of those associations.[100]

The identification of yellow flags is important and requires a shift in the focus of care.

Identify the presence of a treatable lesion – somatic dysfunction

A number of treatment models use elements of T-A-R-T as the basis for the selection of manipulative techniques including HVLA thrust techniques.[11,12,14,21,101,102] The authors advocate that the current convention for the diagnosis of somatic dysfunction T-A-R-T should be expanded to include patient feedback relating to pain provocation and the reproduction of familiar symptoms. Somatic dysfunction is identified by the S-T-A-R-T of diagnosis and is made on the basis of a number of positive findings relating to symptom reproduction, tissue tenderness, asymmetry, range of motion and tissue texture changes (Box 6.4).

Decide upon appropriate intervention

There is research evidence demonstrating the effects of HVLA thrust techniques in increasing range of motion,[37–45] altering pain perception,[40,103,104] reducing pain[105] and altering autonomic reflex activity.[106] However, the rationale for the use of these techniques should also be informed by research showing evidence of efficacy.

Broadly speaking, manipulative techniques should be selected based upon research evidence, practice-based evidence, patient preference and the practitioner's training and experience in the delivery of HVLA thrust techniques.

Research evidence

Research evidence supports the use of spinal manipulation in cervicogenic headache, mechanical neck pain and in patients suffering with acute and chronic mechanical low back pain. Clinical prediction rules allow practitioners to identify sub-groups of patients that are likely to positively respond to spinal manipulation.

Practice-based evidence

Spinal manipulation is a therapeutic intervention that has been used by various cultures and whose use has been documented over time dating from Hippocrates. Spinal manipulation remains one of the most commonly used osteopathic manipulative treatment techniques.[107]

Patient preference

Although research and practice-based evidence support the use of spinal manipulation in the hands of appropriately trained and experienced practitioners, some patients will express a preference for alternative treatment techniques. Conversely other patients who have had a positive response to spinal manipulation will commonly express a preference for HVLA thrust techniques to be used in treatment.

Practitioner training and experience

The key to safety is dependent upon appropriate training, a thorough patient history and physical assessment prior to the application of any manipulative procedure. Appropriate training in the use of HVLA thrust techniques and subsequent skill refinement through regular practice are key elements for safe practice and professional competence.[108]

In clinical practice, the treatment of spinal pain and dysfunction commonly combines several interventions, such as manipulation, mobilization and exercise with evidence supporting a multi-modal approach.[109–112] There is currently no evidence to guide the clinician with regard to the following aspects of manipulative treatment interventions:

1. Which HVLA thrust technique to use.
2. How specific we need to be.
3. Direction of thrust needed.
4. The combination of manual therapy techniques that will be most effective.
5. The most effective sequencing of technique within a multi-modal approach.

In the absence of research evidence, the decision regarding these aspects of treatment can only be made upon the basis of convention and practitioner training and experience.

CONCLUSION

Practitioners rely upon theoretical and clinical models to justify the use of HVLA thrust techniques in clinical practice. Best practice also requires incorporating the results from clinical and epidemiological research with the individual clinical experience and expertise of the practitioner while taking account of patient preferences. Osteopaths have used HVLA thrust techniques for the treatment of somatic dysfunction for many years with increasing research evidence to support the use of these techniques in clinical practice. Clinical decision making relating to the use of these techniques requires the identification and exclusion of red flags, recognition of the impact of yellow flags upon patient presentation and prognosis, the identification of a treatable lesion, patient preference and analysis of benefits versus risk. The treatment of spinal pain and dysfunction commonly combines several interventions e.g. manipulation, mobilization and exercise with evidence supporting a multi-modal approach.

References

1 Kenna C, Murtagh J. Back Pain and Spinal Manipulation, 2nd edn. Oxford: Butterworth-Heinemann; 1989.

2 Bruckner P, Khan K. Clinical Sports Medicine. New York, NY: McGraw-Hill; 1994.

3 Lewit K. Manipulative Therapy in Rehabilitation of the Locomotor System, 2nd edn. Oxford: Butterworth-Heinemann; 1991.

4 Maigne R. Diagnosis and Treatment of Pain of Vertebral Origin. Baltimore, MD: Williams & Wilkins; 1996.

5 Brodeur R. The audible release associated with joint manipulation. J Manipulative Physiol Ther 1995;18(3):155–164.

6 Eder M, Tilscher H. Chiropractic Therapy. Diagnosis and Treatment. Gaithersburg, MD: Aspen; 1990.

7 Sammut E, Searle-Barnes P. Osteopathic Diagnosis. Cheltenham: Stanley Thornes; 1998.

8 Gainsbury J. High-velocity thrust and pathophysiology of segmental dysfunction. In: Glasgow E, Twomey L, Sculle E, et al 1985. Aspects of Manipulative Therapy, 2nd edn. Melbourne: Churchill Livingstone; 1985:Ch. 13.

9 Zusman M. What does manipulation do? The need for basic research. In: Boyling J, Palastanga M eds. 1994. Grieve's Modern Manual Therapy, 2nd edn. New York: Churchill Livingstone; 1994: Ch. 47.

10 Kuchera W, Kuchera M. Osteopathic Principles in Practice. Kirksville, MO: KCOM; 1992.

11 Kappler R, Jones J. Thrust (high-velocity / low-amplitude) techniques. In: Ward R ed. 2003. Foundations for Osteopathic Medicine. Philadelphia: Lippincott Williams & Wilkins; 2003:Ch. 56.

12 Bourdillon J, Day E, Bookhout M. Spinal Manipulation, 5th edn. Oxford: Butterworth-Heinemann; 1992.

13 Kimberly P. Formulating a prescription for osteopathic manipulative treatment. In: Beal M ed. 1992. The Principles of Palpatory Diagnosis and Manipulative Technique. Newark, NJ: American Academy of Osteopathy; 146–152.

14 Greenman PE. Principles of Manual Medicine, 3rd edn. Philadelphia, PA: Lippincott Williams & Wilkins; 2003.

15 Nyberg R, Basmajian J. Rationale for the use of spinal manipulation. In: Basmajian J, Nyberg R eds. 1993. Rational Manual Therapies. Baltimore, MD: Williams & Wilkins; 1993:Ch. 17.

16 Bogduk N, Twomey L. Clinical Anatomy of the Lumbar Spine, 2nd edn. Melbourne: Churchill Livingstone; 1991.

17 Stoddard A. Manual of Osteopathic Practice. London: Hutchinson; 1969.

18 Cyriax J. Textbook of Orthopaedic Medicine1975;Vol1:London: Baillière Tindall; 1975.

19 Terrett A, Vernon H. Manipulation and pain tolerance. A controlled study on the effect of spinal manipulation on paraspinal cutaneous pain tolerance levels. Am J Phys Med 1984;63:217–225.

20 Hoehler F, Tobis J, Buerger A. Spinal manipulation for low back pain. J Am Med Assoc 1981;245:1835–1838.

21 Kuchera W, Kuchera M. Osteopathic Principles in Practice. OH: Greyden Press; 1994:292.

22 Neumann H. Introduction to Manual Medicine. Berlin: Springer; 1989.

23 Fisk J. A controlled trial of manipulation in a selected group of patients with low back pain favouring one side. N Z Med J 1979;90:288–291.

24 Vernon H, Dharmi I, Howley T, et al. Spinal manipulation and beta-endorphin: a controlled study of the effect of a spinal manipulation on plasma beta-endorphin levels in normal males. J Manipulative Physiol Ther 1986;9: 115–123.

25 Flynn T, Fritz J, Whitman J, et al. A clinical prediction rule for classifying patients with low back pain who demonstrate short term improvement with spinal manipulation. Spine 2002;27(24):2835–2843.

26 Childs J, Fritz J, Flynn T, et al. A clinical prediction rule to identify patients with low back pain most likely to benefit from spinal manipulation: A validation study. Ann Intern Med 2004;141 (12):920–928.

27 Tseng Y, Wang W, Chen W, et al. Predictors for the immediate responders to cervical manipulation in patients with neck pain. Man Ther 2006;11 (4):306–315.

28 Cleland J, Childs J, Fritz J, et al. Development of a clinical prediction rule for guiding treatment of a subgroup of patients with neck pain: Use of thoracic spine manipulation, exercise, and patient education. Phys Ther 2007;87(1):9–23.

29 Roston J, Haines R. Cracking in the metacarpophalangeal joint. J Anat 1947;81:165–173.

30 Unsworth A, Dowson D, Wright V. Cracking joints: a bioengineering study of cavitation in the metacarpophalangeal joint. Ann Rheum Dis 1972;30:348–358.

31 Meal G, Scott R. Analysis of the joint crack by simultaneous recording of sound and tension. J Manipulative Physiol Ther 1986;9:189–195.

32 Watson P, Mollan R. Cineradiography of a cracking joint. Br J Radiol 1990;63:145–147.

33 Mierau D, Cassidy J, Bowen V, et al. Manipulation and mobilization of the third metacarpophalangeal joint: a quantitative radiographic and range of motion study. Man Med 1988;3:135–140.

34 Bereznick D, Pecora C, Ross J, et al. The refractory period of the audible 'crack' after lumbar manipulation: A preliminary study. J Manipulative Physiol Ther 2008;31 (3):199–203.

35 Cramer G, Gregerson D, Knudsen J, et al. The effects of side-posture positioning and spinal adjusting on the lumbar Z joints. Spine 2002;27 (22):2459–2466.

36 Cascioli V, Corr P, Till A. An investigation into the production of intra-articular gas bubbles and increase in joint space in the zygapophysial joints of the cervical spine in asymptomatic subjects after spinal manipulation. J Manipulative Physiol Ther 2003;26(6):356–364.

37 Howe DH, Newcombe RG, Wade MT. Manipulation of the cervical spine: a pilot study. J R Coll Gen Pract 1983;33(254):574–579.

38 Nansel D, Cremata E, Carlson J, et al. Effect of unilateral spinal adjustments on goniometrically assessed cervical lateral-flexion end-range asymmetries in otherwise asymptomatic subjects. J Manipulative Physiol Ther 1989;12 (6):419–427.

39 Nansel D, Peneff A, Carlson J, et al. Time course considerations for the effects of unilateral lower cervical adjustments with respect to the amelioration of cervical lateral-flexion passive end-range asymmetry. J Manipulative Physiol Ther 1990;13(6):297–304.

40 Cassidy JD, Quon JA, Lafrance LJ, et al. The effect of manipulation on pain and range of motion in the cervical spine: a pilot study. J Manipulative Physiol Ther 1992;15(8):495–500.

41 Nansel D, Peneff A, Quitoriano D. Effectiveness of upper versus lower cervical adjustments with respect to the amelioration of passive rotational versus lateral-flexion end-range asymmetries in otherwise asymptomatic subjects. J Manipulative Physiol Ther 1992;15(2):99–105.

42 Nilsson N, Christenson HW, Hartrigson J. Lasting changes in passive range of motion after spinal manipulation: a randomised, blind, controlled trial. J Manipulative Physiol Ther 1996;19 (3):165–168.

43 Surkitt D, Gibbons P, McLaughlin P. High velocity low amplitude manipulation of the atlanto-axial joint: Effect on atlanto-axial and cervical spine rotation asymmetry in asymptomatic subjects. J Osteopath Med 2000;3 (1):13–19.

44 Clements B, Gibbons P, McLaughlin P. The amelioration of atlanto-axial asymmetry using high velocity low amplitude manipulation: Is the direction of thrust important? J Osteopath Med 2001;4(1):8–14.

45 Martinez-Segura R, Fernadez-de-la Penas C, et al. Immediate effects on neck pain and active range of motion after a single cervical high velocity low amplitude manipulation in subjects presenting with mechanical neck pain: A randomized controlled trial. J Manipulative Physiol Ther 2006;29(7):511–517.

46 Stodolny J, Chmielewski H. Manual therapy in the treatment of patients with cervical migraine. Man Med 1989;4:49–51.

47 Nordemar R, Thorner C. Treatment of acute cervical pain: a comparative group study. Pain 1981;10:93–101.

48 Flynn T, Fritz J, Wainner R, et al. The audible pop is not necessary for successful spinal high-velocity thrust manipulation in individuals with low back pain. Arch Phys Med Rehabil 2003;84:1057–1060.

49 Flynn T, Childs J, Fritz J. The audible pop from high-velocity thrust manipulation and outcome in individuals with low back pain. J Manipulative Physiol Ther 2006;29(1):40–45.

50 Reggars J, Pollard H. Analysis of zygapophysial joint cracking during chiropractic manipulation. J Manipulative Physiol Ther 1995;18(2):65–71.

51 Beffa R, Mathews R. Does the adjustment cavitate the targeted joint? An investigation into the

location of cavitation sounds. J Manipulative Physiol Ther 2004;27(2):e2.

52 Ross J, Bereznick D, McGill S. Determining cavitation location during lumbar and thoracic spinal manipulation. Is spinal manipulation accurate and specific? Spine 2004;29 (13):1452–1457.

53 Bolton A, Moran R, Standen C. An investigation into the side of joint cavitation associated with cervical spine manipulation. Int J Osteopath Med 2007;10(4):88–96.

54 Swezey R, Swezey S. The consequences of habitual knuckle cracking. West J Med 1975;122:377–379.

55 Castellanos J, Axelrod D. Effect of habitual knuckle cracking on hand function. Ann Rheum Dis 1990;49:308–309.

56 Sackett D, Richardson W, Rosenberg W, et al. Evidence Based Medicine. How to Practice & Teach EBM. New York: Churchill Livingstone; 1997.

57 Pedersen T, Gluud C, Gotzsche P, et al. What is evidence-based medicine? Ugeskr Laeg 2001;163 (27):3769–3772.

58 Bronfort G, Hass M, Evans R, et al. Efficacy of spinal manipulation and mobilization for low back and neck pain: A systematic review and best evidence synthesis. Spine 2004;4(3):335–356.

59 Koes B, Assendelft W, Heijden G, et al. Spinal manipulation for low back pain. An updated systematic review of randomized clinical trials. Spine 1996;21(24):2860–2871.

60 van Tulder M, Koes B, Bouter L. Conservative treatment of acute and chronic nonspecific low back pain. A systematic review of randomized controlled trials of the most common interventions. Spine 1997;22(18):2128–2156.

61 Bronfort G. Spinal manipulation: current state of research and its indications. Neurol Clin 1999;17 (1):91–111.

62 Ferreira M, Ferreira P, Latimer J, et al. Does spinal manipulative therapy help people with chronic low back pain? Aust J Physiother 2002;48 (4):277–284.

63 Pengel H, Maher C, Refshauge K. Systematic review of conservative interventions for subacute low back pain. Clin Rehabil 2002;16 (8):811–820.

64 Cherkin D, Sherman K, Deyo R, et al. A review of the evidence for the effectiveness, safety, and cost of acupuncture, massage therapy, and spinal manipulation for back pain. Ann Intern Med 2003;138(11):898–906.

65 Ferreira M, Ferreira P, Latimer J, et al. Efficacy of spinal manipulative therapy for low back pain of less than three months' duration. J Manipulative Physiol Ther 2003;26(9):593–601.

66 Willem J, Assendelft W, Morton S, et al. Spinal manipulative therapy for low back pain. A meta-analysis of effectiveness relative to other therapies. Ann Intern Med 2003;138 (11):871–881.

67 Assendelft W, Morton S, Yu E, et al. Spinal manipulative therapy for low back pain. Cochrane Database Syst Rev 2004;1:CD000447.

68 Van Tulder M, Koes B, Malmivaara A. Outcome of non-invasive treatment modalities on back pain: an evidence review. Eur Spine J 2006;15 (Suppl 1):S64–S81.

69 Bronfort G, Haas M, Evans R, et al. Evidence-informed management of chronic low back pain with spinal manipulation and mobilization. Spine J 2008;8(1):213–225.

70 Mior S. Manipulation and mobilization in the treatment of chronic pain. Clin J Pain 2001;17 (4):S70–S76.

71 Bronfort G, Haas M, Evans R, et al. Efficacy of spinal manipulation and mobilization for low back pain and neck pain: a systematic review and best evidence synthesis. Spine J 2004;4 (3):335–356.

72 Hurwitz E, Aker P, Adams A, et al. Manipulation and mobilization of the cervical spine. A systematic review of the literature. Spine 1996;21 (15):1746–1759.

73 Gross A, Kay T, Hondras M, et al. Manual therapy for mechanical neck disorders: a systematic review. Man Ther 2002;7(3):131–149.

74 Gross A, Hoving J, Haines T, et al. A Cochrane review of manipulation and mobilization for mechanical neck disorders. Spine 2004;29 (14):1541–1548.

75 Vernon H, Humphreys K, Hagino C. Chronic mechanical neck pain in adults treated by manual therapy: A systematic review of change scores in randomized clinical trials. J Manipulative Physiol Ther 2007;30(3):215–227.

76 Hurwitz E, Carragee E, van der Velde G, et al. Treatment of neck pain: Non-invasive interventions. Results of the bone and joint decade 2000-2010 task force on neck pain and its associated disorders. Spine 2008; (4S): S123–S152.

77 Bronfort G, Assendelft W, Evans R, et al. Efficacy of spinal manipulation for chronic headache: a systematic review. J Manipulative Physiol Ther 2001;24(7):457–466.

78 Waddell G. The Back Pain Revolution, 2nd edn. Edinburgh, UK: Churchill Livingstone; 2004.

79 UK BEAM Trial Team. United Kingdom Back Pain Exercise and Manipulation (UK BEAM) randomised trial: Effectiveness of physical treatments for back pain in primary care. BMJ 2004;329(7479):1377.

80 UK BEAM Trial Team. United Kingdom back pain exercise and manipulation (UK BEAM) randomised trial: cost effectiveness of physical treatments for back pain in primary care. BMJ 2004;329(7479):1381:Epub.

81 Chou R, Qaseem A, Snow V, et al. Diagnosis and treatment of low back pain: A joint clinical practice guideline from the American College of Physicians and the American Pain Society. Ann Intern Med 2007;147(7):478–491.

82 Brennan G, Fritz J, Hunter S, et al. Identifying subgroups of patients with acute / subacute non specific low back pain. Spine 2006;31 (6):623–631.

83 Fritz J, Delitto A, Erhard R. Comparison of classification-based physical therapy with therapy based on clinical practice guidelines for patients with acute low back pain: A randomized clinical trial. Spine 2003;28(13):1363–1371.

84 Childs J, Fritz J, Piva S, et al. Proposal of a classification system for patients with neck pain. J Orthop Sports Phys Ther 2004;34 (11):686–696.

85 O'Sullivan P. Diagnosis and classification of chronic low back pain disorders: Maladaptive movement and motor control impairments as underlying mechanism. Man Ther 2005;10 (4):242–255.

86 Fritz J, Brennan G. Preliminary examination of a proposed treatment-based classification system for patients receiving physical therapy interventions for neck pain. Phys Ther 2007;87 (5):513–524.

87 Billis E, McCarthy C, Oldham J. Subclassification of low back pain: A cross-country comparison. Eur Spine J 2007;16(7):865–879.

88 Fritz J, Cleland J, Childs J. Subgrouping patients with low back pain: Evolution of a classification approach to physical therapy. J Orthop Sports Phys Ther 2007;37(6):290–302.

89 Fritz J, Lindsay W, Matheson J, et al. Is there a subgroup of patients with low back pain likely to benefit from mechanical traction? Results of a randomized clinical trial and subgrouping analysis. Spine 2007;32(26):E793–E800.

90 O'Sullivan P, Beals D. Diagnosis and classification of pelvic girdle pain disorders – Part 1: A mechanism based approach within a biopsychosocial framework. Man Ther 2007;12 (2):86–97.

91 Grotle M, Vollestad N, Veierod M, et al. Fear-avoidance beliefs and distress in relation to disability in acute and chronic low back pain. Pain 2004;112(3):343–352.

92 Steenstra I, Verbeek J, Heymans M, et al. Prognostic factors for duration of sick leave in patients sick listed with acute low back pain: A systematic review of the literature. Occup Environ Med 2005;62(12):851–860.

93 Grotle M, Vollestad N, Brox J. Clinical course and impact of fear-avoidance beliefs in low back pain: Prospective cohort study of acute and chronic low back pain. Spine 2006;31 (9):1038–1046.

94 Iles R, Davidson M, Taylor N. A systematic review of psychosocial predictors of failure to return to work in non-chronic non-specific low back pain. Occup Environ Med 2008;65(8):507–517: Epub.

95 Grotle M, Brox J, Glomsrod B, et al. Prognostic factors in first-time care seekers due to acute low back pain. Eur J Pain 2007;11(3):290–298.

96 Keeley P, Creed F, Tomenson B, et al. Psychosocial predictors of health-related quality of life and health service utilisation in people with chronic low back pain. Pain 2008; 135(1-2):142–150:Epub.

97 Henschke N, Maher C, Refshauge K, et al. Prognosis in patients with recent onset low back pain in Australian primary care: inception cohort study. BMJ 2008;337:a171. doi: 10.1136/bmj. a171 Epub.

98 Carroll L, Hogg-Johnson S, van der Velde G, et al. Course and prognostic factors for neck pain in the general population. Results of the bone and joint decade 2000-2010 Task Force on neck pain and its associated disorders. Spine 2008;33 (4S):S75–S82.

99 Landers M, Creger R, Baker C, et al. The use of fear-avoidance beliefs and nonorganic signs in predicting prolonged disability in patients with neck pain. Man Ther 2008;13(3):239–248.

100 Kent P, Keating J. Can we predict poor recovery from recent-onset nonspecific low back pain? A systematic review. Man Ther 2008;13 (1):12–28.

101 DiGiovanna EL, Schiowitz S. An Osteopathic Approach to Diagnosis and Treatment, 2nd edn. Philadelphia, PA: Lippincott Williams & Wilkins; 1997.

102 Mitchell F. The Muscle Energy Manual. East Lansing, MI: MET; 1995.

103 Vernon H, Aker P, Burns S, et al. Pressure pain threshold evaluation of the effect of spinal manipulation in the treatment of chronic neck pain: A pilot study. J Manipulative Physiol Ther 1990;13(1):285–289.

104 Cleland J, Childs J, McRae M, et al. Immediate effects of thoracic manipulation in patients with neck pain: A randomized clinical trial. Man Ther 2005;10(2):127–135.

105 Fernandez-de-la Penas C, Palomeque-del-Cerro L, Rodriguez-Blanco C, et al. Changes in neck pain and active range of motion after a single thoracic

spine manipulation in subjects presenting with mechanical neck pain: A case series. J Manipulative Physiol Ther 2007;30(4): 312–320.

106 Gibbons P, Gosling C, Holmes M. The short term effects of cervical manipulation on edge light pupil cycle time: a pilot study. J Manipulative Physiol Ther 2000;23(7):465–469.

107 Johnson S, Kurtz M. Osteopathic manipulative treatment techniques preferred by contemporary osteopathic physicians. J Am Osteopath Assoc 2003;103(5):219–224.

108 Vick D, McKay C, Zengerle C. The safety of manipulative treatment: Review of the literature from 1925 to 1993. J Am Osteopath Assoc 1996;96(2):113–115.

109 Jull G, Trott P, Potter H, et al. A randomized controlled trial of exercise and manipulative therapy for cervicogenic headache. Spine 2002;27(17):1835–1843.

110 Gross A, Kay T, Kennedy C, et al. Clinical practice guideline on the use of manipulation or mobilization in the treatment of adults with mechanical neck disorders. Man Ther 2002;7 (4):193–205.

111 Grunnesjo M, Bogefeldt B, Svardsudd K, et al. A randomized controlled clinical trial of stay-active care versus manual therapy in addition to stay-active care: Functional variables and pain. J Manipulative Physiol Ther 2004;27 (7):431–441.

112 Walker M, Boyles R, Young B, et al. The effectiveness of manual physical therapy and exercise for mechanical neck pain. A randomized clinical trial. Spine 2008;33 (22):2371–2378.

7

Validation of clinical practice by research

Responsibility for the scientific credence that can be afforded osteopathic medicine rests largely within its own discipline. The osteopathic profession is obligated to question the value of teaching unsubstantiated doctrines, except within their historical perspective. Students and the profession should be encouraged to engage in active research. Research is needed both to establish the clinical efficacy of osteopathic therapeutic intervention and to elaborate the biological basis and physiological mechanisms that underlie the osteopathic principles of practice. Patient satisfaction is also an important measure of the quality of care.[1] If there is to be a commitment to research, where should the osteopathic profession focus its research funds and activities?

WHY UNDERTAKE RESEARCH?

Given the financial constraints placed upon health expenditure and the increasing pressure upon third-party payers to rationalize and limit costs, health professionals will be required to demonstrate efficacy of treatment. It will no longer be acceptable to claim that therapy is beneficial solely because individual patients report improvement after treatment. The challenge is to demonstrate that symptom improvement is a direct outcome of specific intervention rather than natural recovery and that this intervention is more effective and cost-effective than marketplace competitors. Bogduk[2] argues that research is not an

indulgence of academics, but constitutes the basis of best practice and quality assurance.

Various osteopathic authors have acknowledged the need for research and the importance of continuing to search for new knowledge.[3-8] The need for research should be indisputable, but where should the osteopathic profession's resources be concentrated? Bogduk and Mercer[9] express a view that it is more valuable to demonstrate the efficacy of a therapy before one explores its mechanism. They suggest there may be limited value in utilizing scarce resources researching the underlying mechanisms of a therapy that may eventually be shown to be ineffective.

It would also be reasonable for a profession to hold the view that there is a place for both therapeutic trials and continuing research to explore the biological basis and physiological mechanisms that underpin osteopathic treatment. However, it should be recognized that, even if we had a clear understanding of the biological and physiological mechanisms underlying all osteopathic therapeutic interventions, this in itself would not prove that their use would produce a positive clinical outcome. Only properly conducted clinical trials can legitimize a therapy by demonstrating positive outcomes from therapeutic intervention. Many government bodies, professional associations and third-party payers promote evidence-based guidelines for the management of musculoskeletal pain.[10-15] However, such guidelines are often promoted without evidence of their effectiveness.[16] Willem et al[17] noted that all national guidelines on the management of low back pain included the use of spinal manipulation. However, the data upon which national recommendations are based has been interpreted differently, leading to conflicting guidelines between countries for the use of spinal manipulation in the management of both acute and chronic back pain.

WHERE SHOULD RESEARCH BE FOCUSED?

Research effort should be directed towards designing and implementing effective therapeutic trials that could demonstrate the efficacy or otherwise of therapeutic interventions.[9] Validation of osteopathic practice by outcome studies is essential. Management of patients utilizing outcome measures has the benefit of establishing baselines, documenting progress and assisting in quality assurance.[18]

Osteopathic practice is diverse. Individual practitioners, depending upon their style of practice and interests, treat a wide variety of different complaints. Osteopaths see and treat a significant number of patients presenting with spinal pain.[19,20] Outcome studies on patients presenting with spinal pain and disability are an obvious area for osteopathic research. Despite this fact, there is a paucity of osteopathic outcome studies. The studies that have been published included small patient numbers, variability in methodology and outcomes.[20]

Various authors[4,8,21–23] highlight the point that there are significant difficulties associated with clinical research in the osteopathic area. Stoddard[21] emphasizes that clinical research in osteopathy is hampered by the complexity and diversity of the presenting problems and the difficulties associated with patient allocation to syndrome groups that vary constantly over time. Although there has been a focus upon quantitative research it is increasingly recognized that qualitative research has a distinct and important contribution to make to healthcare research.[24] Qualitative research has not often been used as an evidence resource for systematic reviews.

As individualized patient treatment is complex, research should utilize and value both qualitative and quantitative research methods.[25] However, similar problems associated with clinical research exist for other disciplines practising manual therapies. Despite the difficulties, other disciplines are participating in an increasing number of research projects.

PATIENT CLASSIFICATION

A possible spectrum of research designs would include conventional and unconventional group designs, ethnomethodological designs and single case studies.[26] Each research method has advantages and limitations, with varying applicability, differing ranges of validity and ethical constraints and will generate differing sets of data. Which approach would be most useful for outcome studies in osteopathic medicine? The nature of the research question should guide the selection of research design.

One of the major problems associated with clinical trials related to spinal pain lies in the area of diagnosis. The aetiology of most spinal pain is unknown, with the pathological or structural diagnosis uncertain in the majority of patients. Assessment procedures used may not be able to diagnose the pathology involved or may be incorrectly interpreted. Problems associated with poor inter-observer and intra-observer reliability for clinical findings further confound the picture.

Palpatory findings are integral to the establishment of an osteopathic diagnosis. For palpatory diagnosis to be useful for classification purposes, good reliability needs to be demonstrated. Many studies and systematic reviews indicate that inter- and intra-examiner reliability for palpatory motion testing without pain provocation is poor.[27-38] For these reasons, current osteopathic diagnostic labels cannot be used effectively in clinical trials of spinal pain and disability and an alternative means of classification needs to be identified.

The Quebec Task Force[39] recognized the lack of uniformity in diagnostic terminology

Table 7.1 Classification of activity-related spinal disorders

Classification	Symptoms	Duration of symptoms from onset	Working status at time of evaluation
1	Pain without radiation	a ($<$ 7 days)	
2	Pain + radiation to extremity, proximally	b (7 days–7 weeks)	W (working)
3	Pain + radiation to extremity, distally	c ($>$ 7 weeks)	I (idle)
4	Pain + radiation to upper / lower limb + neurological signs		
5	Presumptive compression of a spinal nerve root on a simple roentgenogram (i.e. spinal instability or fracture)		
6	Compression of a spinal root confirmed by: – specific imaging techniques (i.e. CAT, myelography or MRI) – other diagnostic techniques (e.g. electromyography, venography)		
7	Spinal stenosis		
8	Post-surgical status, 1–6 months after intervention		

9	Post-surgical status, $>$ 6 months after intervention
	   9.1 Asymptomatic
	   9.2 Symptomatic		

10	Chronic pain syndrome		W (working)
11	Other diagnoses		I (idle)

Source: Quebec Task Force.[39]

used for spinal disorders and proposed a classification that did not depend upon pathological entities, but reflected the clinical presentations encountered in practice. A modified form of this classification has been utilized for conducting research. This classification system had the merit of enabling clinicians, regardless of discipline, to categorize patients with spinal pain in the clinical setting and it links patient symptomatology with duration of symptoms and working status (Table 7.1). The Quebec Task Force classification consisted of 11 categories with classification based upon historical markers and clinical and paraclinical examinations. Some categories were further subdivided by stage (i.e. acute, subacute and chronic) and whether the patient is able to work.

Some authors suggested different methods of patient classification.[40,41] DeRosa and Porterfield[41] modified the Quebec Task Force classification for spinal pain, making it more appropriate for physical therapy diagnosis (Table 7.2).

Categorizing patients using the Quebec Task Force or a similar system of classification enabled outcome studies to be performed on groups of patients with spinal pain without the need for a specific osteopathic or mechanical diagnosis. This did not obviate the need for the practitioner to undertake a full and thorough assessment of each patient, but allowed classification of patients into groups for the purpose of research. This form of classification removed some of the obstacles to research associated with a lack of standardization

Table 7.2 Modified physical therapy diagnosis classification

Category	Definition
1	Back pain without radiation
2	Back pain with referral to extremity, proximally
3	Back pain with referral to extremity, distally
4	Extremity pain greater than back pain
5	Back pain with radiation and neurological signs
6	Post-surgical status ($<$ 6 months or $>$ 6 months)
7	Chronic pain syndrome

Source: DeRosa and Porterfield.[41]

and validation of diagnostic terminology in spinal disorders.

The Quebec Task Force[42] published a similar classification for whiplash-associated disorders. This classification was said to 'provide, categories that are jointly exhaustive and mutually exclusive, clinically meaningful, stand the test of common sense and are "user friendly" to investigators, clinicians, and patients'. This classification system allowed outcome studies on 'whiplash' patients to be undertaken.

These classification systems enabled patients to be placed into discrete sub-groups. A study by Brennan et al reported that practitioners demonstrated an ability, using signs and symptoms, to identify sub-groups of patients with low back pain and then match them to specific treatment approaches. Those patients matched by the practitioner to specific interventions showed statistically significant improvement when compared with non-matched controls.[43] This indicates that within any population of spinal pain patients there are sub-groups of patients who are likely to respond better to one intervention than another and that practitioners have an ability to identify likely positive responders. Several classification systems for spinal and pelvic girdle pain have now been developed in an attempt to identify sub-groups of patients who are likely to respond positively to specific interventions.[44-51]

Are there historical and clinical features that would identify positive responders from non-responders to high-velocity low-amplitude (HVLA) thrust techniques? Research into the predictive value of specific clinical findings to identify patients with spinal pain who are likely to benefit from spinal manipulation has led to the development of clinical prediction rules. Clinical prediction rules consist of combinations of variables obtained from self-report measures, patient history and examination that assist in identifying those patients with spinal pain most likely to respond to spinal manipulation.[52-55]

MEASURING OUTCOMES

Consideration needs to be given as to what instruments might be used to measure patient outcomes arising from osteopathic intervention. The process of selecting appropriate measuring instruments can be broken down into three stages:

1. The researcher must identify what he or she wishes to measure, e.g. spinal pain and disability.
2. What is to be measured must be defined in quantifiable terms, e.g. the intensity of pain suffered by the patient, the impact the pain and disability have upon the patient's activities of daily living and work, etc.
3. Selection of appropriate data collection and recording instruments that will give reliable and valid results.

Broadly speaking, outcome measures attempt to quantify pain, physical impairment, limitation of activity, impact upon work and

Table 7.3 A proposed set of patient-based outcome measures for use in spinal disorders

Domain	Instrument
Back specific function	Roland–Morris or Oswestry
Generic health status	SF-36 version 2.0
Pain	Bodily pain scale of SF-36
	(optional) Chronic Pain Grade
Work disability	Work status
Satisfaction: back specific	Days off work and days of cut down work
	Time to return to work
	Satisfaction with care: Patient Satisfaction Scale
	Satisfaction with treatment outcome: Global question

Source: Adapted from Bombardier.[56]

leisure and psychosocial factors. It is recommended that a full evaluation of spinal disorders should include a disability measure, a general health measure, a pain scale, a measure of employment and a measure of patient satisfaction (Table 7.3).[56] Although patient records are easily accessible to the practitioner, there are problems associated with this form of data collection for the purpose of outcomes assessment. Recording in patient records lacks standardization and is often incomplete and what is recorded may not reflect what has actually occurred. Practitioners also record physical examination findings, but the large variability in normal values and poor inter-examiner agreement limit the use of such tests in research.

A variety of easily used tools has been developed that allow practitioners to assess specific outcomes resulting from therapeutic interventions. Liebenson and Yeomans[18] identified eight categories of available outcome approaches (Table 7.4). Additional validated measurement instruments have been developed over time.

As the range of questionnaires and pain-rating scales is diverse, researchers must be confident that they have selected the most appropriate measurement tools for their clinical trials. A different approach and rating instrument would be selected for assessment of chronic spinal pain, with the possibility of a strong affective component compared with acute spinal pain. Clinicians undertaking research must be cognizant of both the advantages and disadvantages of individual outcome assessment instruments. Once the most appropriate measurement tools have been selected, they should be used throughout the period of the study. Different scales and questionnaires are not interchangeable.

Specific questionnaires can measure a patient's presenting level of pain and disability and be used to reflect changes in that pain and disability after treatment and over time. The Oswestry Low Back Pain Disability Questionnaire[57-59] and the Roland–Morris Low Back Pain Disability Questionnaire[60] have been shown in randomized controlled trials to have both validity and reliability in measuring results for patients with back pain. A modified Oswestry Low Back Pain Disability Questionnaire demonstrated superior measurement properties and higher levels of test–retest reliability and responsiveness compared with the Quebec Back Pain Disability Scale.[61] The Likert modified version of the Roland–Morris Disability Questionnaire has shown greater sensitivity to change over time than the original version.[62] Vernon and Mior[63] demonstrated a high degree of test–retest reliability and internal consistency for the Neck Disability Index. This index was modified from the Oswestry Low Back Pain Disability Questionnaire. A whiplash-specific disability questionnaire has also been developed that has shown internal consistency and validity.[64]

73

Table 7.4 Outcome approaches

Category based on assessment goals	Outcomes assessment instrument
1. Pain level	1 Numerical pain scale (NPS)
	2 Visual analogue scale (VAS)
	3 McGill / Melzack Pain Questionnaire
2. Region / condition-specific disability questionnaires	4 Oswestry Low Back Pain Disability Questionnaire
	5 Roland–Morris Low Back Pain Disability Questionnaire
LBP	6 Dallas Pain Questionnaire
Neck	7 Low Back Pain 'TyPE'
Headache	8 Neck Disability Index (NDI)
	9 Headache Disability Index (HDI)
3. General health	10 Dartmouth COOP charts
	11 Health Status Questionnaire 2.0
	12 Short Form (SF)-36
4. Psychometrics	13 Health Status Questionnaire (HSQ) 20
	14 SF-16
	15 Waddell's Non-organic LBP signs
	16 Modified Zung Questionnaire
	17 Modified Somatic Perception Questionnaire
	18 Beck's Depression Scale
	19 Fear Avoidance Beliefs Questionnaire
	20 SCL-90-R
5. Patient satisfaction	21 Patient Satisfaction Questionnaire
	22 Visit Specific Questionnaire
	23 Chiropractic Satisfaction Questionnaire
6. Job dissatisfaction	24 APGAR
7. General disability	25 Vermont Disability Questionnaire
	26 Vermont Disability Questionnaire: brief form
	27 Functional Assessment Screening Questionnaire
	28 Fear Avoidance Beliefs Questionnaire
8. Job demands	29 Job Demands Questionnaire

Source: Adapted from Liebenson and Yeomans.[18]

These questionnaires have been demonstrated to reliably detect changes in the level of disability and impairment over time and are reproducible and acceptable to patients. Some questionnaires include items that may not be directly relevant to a particular patient. The patient-specific functional questionnaire allows the measurement of patient-generated and specific activities that are of concern to them.[65,66]

The subjective sensation of pain can be self-rated by patients using a number of different measures. The most commonly used include the visual analogue scale, numerical rating scale and the verbal rating scale. With the visual analogue scale, the patient records the level of pain by making a single perpendicular line along a 100 mm scale (Fig. 7.1). This can be repeated at second and subsequent visits. The researcher measures the pain level for all visits by measuring from the left end of the 100 mm line. As the line is 100 mm long, all measurements can be expressed as a percentage. However, even with this simple scale, experience has demonstrated that patients need oral reinforcement and supervision in addition to written instructions in case they use a circle or a cross to indicate

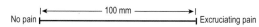

Figure 7.1 Visual analogue scale.

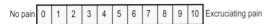

Figure 7.2 Numerical rating scale.

level of pain rather than a perpendicular line. Such responses would render the rating imprecise and invalid.

The numerical rating scale is similar to the visual analogue scale, but offers the patient more defined pain categories to mark. The patient is asked to rate the severity of pain by marking one box on the scale in Figure 7.2.

With the verbal rating scale, the patient must select an adjective, from a standardized list, that best describes the pain. There are many verbal rating scales with the level of pain severity being represented in the questionnaire varying from as few as 4 up to 14 (Fig. 7.3).

Not noticeable	
Just noticeable	
Very weak	
Weak	
Mild	
Moderate	
Strong	
Very strong	
Intense	
Very intense	
Severe	
Excruciating	

Figure 7.3 Twelve-point verbal rating scale.

There is evidence that tissue tenderness is also measurable. The American College of Rheumatology recommends a five-grade classification of tenderness (Box 7.1).[67]

Many practitioners will encounter patients with chronic spinal pain in clinical practice. It is now recognized that a biopsychosocial model is useful in helping manage these patients.[68] The Distress and Risk Assessment Method (DRAM) has been developed as an easily applied and non-threatening tool that allows a practitioner to determine whether a patient requires a more comprehensive psychological evaluation.[69] Questionnaires measuring depression and other mood states are available but have been criticized as they

Box 7.1 Standardized palpation of tenderness

Using 4 kg of pressure (enough to blanch the tip of the thumbnail if you pressed on a table):

Grade 0   No tenderness
Grade I   Tenderness with no physical response
Grade II   Tenderness with grimace and / or flinch
Grade III   Tenderness with withdrawal (+ jump sign)
Grade IV   Withdrawal to non-noxious stimuli

(*Source*: Wolfe et al.[67])

were not developed in patient populations suffering from chronic pain. The Depression, Anxiety and Positive Outlook Scale (DAPOS) has been developed in an attempt to measure these factors in patients that present with chronic pain.[70]

CONCLUSION

There is a need for the osteopathic profession to undertake clinical research. Establishing the efficacy of osteopathic management was rated highly in a study of responses from a group of osteopathic professionals.[71] Structured questionnaires and pain-rating scales have been shown to be valid and reliable research instruments to evaluate the efficacy of any given therapy in altering pain and disability. Biopsychosocial factors are of significance in the management of patients with chronic spinal pain and questionnaires allow quantification of these factors. The use of standardized classification systems enables comparison of efficacy of treatment between professions and of therapeutic approaches within a profession. The development of clinical prediction rules will assist in identifying those patients with spinal pain most likely to respond to spinal manipulation. As osteopathic treatment is a complex and integrated intervention, research should utilize and value both qualitative and quantitative research methods.

References

1 Donabedian A. The quality of care: how can it be assessed? J Am Med Assoc 1988;260:1743–1748.

2 Bogduk N, Editorial. Scientific monograph of the Quebec Task Force on whiplash-associated disorders. Spine 1995;20(8S):8–9.

3 Moor D. Aspects of clinical research in osteopathy. Aust J Osteopathy 1992;5(1):6–14.

4 Ward RC. Myofascial release concepts. In: Basmajian J V, Nyberg R eds. Rational Manual Therapies. Baltimore, MD: Williams & Wilkins; 1993:223–241.

5 Spaltro K. Northup and Jokl speeches round out research conference. DO 1984;24:81–82.

6 Howell J. The paradox of osteopathy. N Engl J Med 1999;341(19):1465–1468.

7 Lucas N, Moran R. Researching osteopathy: Who is responsible? Int J Osteopath Med 2007; 10(2–3):33–35.

8 Leach J. Towards an osteopathic understanding of evidence. Int J Osteopath Med 2008;11(1):3–6.

9 Bogduk N, Mercer S. Selection and application of treatment. In: Refshauge K, Gass E eds. Musculoskeletal Physiotherapy, 1st edn. Oxford: Butterworth-Heinemann; 1995:169–181.

10 National Health and Medical Research Council (NHMRC). Evidence Based Management of Acute Musculoskeletal Pain. National Health and Medical Research Council; 2003:http://www.nhmrc.gov.au/publications/synopses/cp94syn.htm.

11 Gross A, Kay T, Kennedy C, et al. Clinical practice guidelines on the use of manipulation or mobilization in the treatment of adults with mechanical neck disorders. Man Ther 2002;7 (4):193–205.

12 Chou R, Qaseem A, Snow V, et al. Diagnosis and treatment of low back pain: A joint clinical practice guideline from the American College of Physicians and the American Pain Society. Ann Intern Med 2007;147(7):478–491.

13 Chou R, Huffman L. American Pain Society, American College of Physicians. Nonpharmacologic therapies for acute and chronic low back pain: a review of the evidence for an American Pain Society / American College of Physician's clinical practice guideline. Ann Intern Med 2007;147(7):492–504.

14 Motor Accidents Authority NSW. Guidelines for the management of acute whiplash-associated disorders, 2nd edn. 2007:www.maa.nsw.gov.au.

15 Vleeming A, Albert H, Ostgaard H, et al. European guidelines for the diagnosis and treatment of pelvic girdle pain. Eur Spine J 2008;17 (6):794–819.

16 McGuirk B, King W, Govind J, et al. Safety, efficacy, and cost effectiveness of evidence-based guidelines for the management of acute low back pain in primary care. Spine 2001;26 (23):2615–2622.

17 Willem J, Assendelft W, Morton S, et al. Spinal manipulative therapy for low back pain. A meta-analysis of effectiveness relative to other therapies. Ann Intern Med 2003;138 (11):871–881.

18 Liebenson C, Yeomans S. Outcomes assessment in musculoskeletal medicine. Man Ther 1997;2 (2):67–74.

19 Licciardone J, Herron K. Characteristics, satisfaction, and perceptions of patients receiving ambulatory healthcare from osteopathic physicians: A comparative national survey. J Am Osteopath Assoc 2001;101(7):374–385.

20 Licciardone J, King H, Hensel K, et al. Osteopathic health outcomes in chronic low back pain: The osteopathic trial. Osteopath Med Prim Care 2008; Apr 25; 2:5. Online. Available: http://www.om-pc.com/content/2/1/5.

21 Stoddard A. Manual of Osteopathic Practice. London: Hutchinson Medical; 1969:281–282.

22 Keating JC, Seville J, Meeker WC, et al. Intrasubject experimental designs in osteopathic medicine: Applications in clinical practice. In: Beal M C ed. The Principles of Palpatory Diagnosis and Manipulative Technique. Newark, NJ: American Academy of Osteopathy; 1990:205–214.

23 Licciardone J, Russo D. Blinding protocols, treatment credibility, and expectancy; Methodological issues in clinical trials of osteopathic manipulative treatment. J Am Osteopath Assoc 2006;106(8):457–463.

24 Dixon-Woods M, Fitzpatrick R, Roberts K. Including qualitative research in systematic reviews: Opportunities and problems. J Eval Clin Pract 2008;7(2):125–133.

25 Verhoef M, Lewith G, Ritenbaugh C, et al. Complementary and alternative medicine whole systems research: Beyond identification of inadequacies of the RCT. Complement Ther Med 2005;13(3):206–212.

26 Aldridge D. Single-case research designs. Complement Med Res 1988;3(1):37–46.

27 Van Duersen LLJM, Patijn J, Ockhuysen AL, et al. The value of some clinical tests of the sacroiliac joint. Man Med 1990;5:96–99.

28 Laslett M, Williams M. The reliability of selected pain provocation tests for sacroiliac joint pathology. In: Leeming A, Mooney V, Dorman T, et al. eds. The Integrated Function of the Lumbar Spine and Sacroiliac Joint. Rotterdam: ECO; 1995:485–498.

29 Gonnella C, Paris S, Kutner M. Reliability in evaluating passive intervertebral motion. Phys Ther 1982;62:436–444.

30 Matyas T, Bach T. The reliability of selected techniques in clinical arthrokinematics. Aust J Physiother 1985;31(5):175–195.

31 Harvey D, Byfield D. Preliminary studies with a mechanical model for the evaluation of spinal motion palpation. Clin Biomechanics 1991;6:79–82.

32 Lewit K, Liebenson C. Palpation – problems and implications. J Manipulative Physiol Ther 1993;16 (9):586–590.

33 Panzer DM. The reliability of lumbar motion palpation. J Manipulative Physiol Ther 1992;15 (8):518–524.

34 Love RM, Brodeur R. Inter- and intra-examiner reliability of motion palpation for the thoracolumbar spine. J Manipulative Physiol Ther 1987;10(1):1–4.

35 Smedmark V, Wallin M, Arvidsson I. Inter-examiner reliability in assessing passive intervertebral motion of the cervical spine. Man Ther 2000;5(2):97–101.

36 Hestboek L, Leboeuf-Yde C. Are chiropractic tests for the lumbo-pelvic spine reliable and valid? A systematic critical literature review. J Manipulative Physiol Ther 2000;23(4):258–275.

37 Van Trijffel E, Anderegg Q, Bossuyt P, et al. Inter-examiner reliability of passive assessment of intervertebral motion in the cervical and lumbar spine: A systematic review. Man Ther 2005;10 (4):256–269.

38 Robinson H, Brox J, Robinson R, et al. The reliability of selected motion and pain provocation tests for the sacroiliac joint. Man Ther 2007;12 (1):72–79.

39 Force QT. Scientific approach to the assessment and management of activity-related spinal disorders. Spine 1987;12(7S):16–21.

40 Deyo RA. Clinical Concepts in Regional Musculo-skeletal Illness. London: Grune & Stratton; 1987:25–50.

41 DeRosa CP, Porterfield JA. A physical therapy model for the treatment of low back pain. Phys Ther 1992;72(4):261–269.

42 Force QT. Scientific monograph of the Quebec Task Force on whiplash-associated disorders: redefining 'whiplash' and its management. Spine 1995;20(8S):10–73.

43 Brennan G, Fritz J, Hunter S, et al. Identifying subgroups of patients with acute / subacute non specific low back pain. Spine 2006;31(6):623–631.

44 Fritz J, Delitto A, Erhard R. Comparison of classification-based physical therapy with therapy based on clinical practice guidelines for patients with acute low back pain: A randomized clinical trial. Spine 2003;28(13):1363–1371.

45 Childs J, Fritz J, Piva S, et al. Proposal of a classification system for patients with neck pain.

J Orthop Sports Phys Ther 2004;34(11): 686–696.

46 O'Sullivan P. Diagnosis and classification of chronic low back pain disorders: Maladaptive movement and motor control impairments as underlying mechanism. Man Ther 2005;10 (4):242–255.

47 Fritz J, Brennan G. Preliminary examination of a proposed treatment-based classification system for patients receiving physical therapy interventions for neck pain. Phys Ther 2007;87 (5):513–524.

48 Billis E, McCarthy C, Oldham J. Subclassification of low back pain: A cross-country comparison. Eur Spine J 2007;16(7):865–879.

49 Fritz J, Cleland J, Childs J. Subgrouping patients with low back pain: Evolution of a classification approach to physical therapy. J Orthop Sports Phys Ther 2007;37(6):290–302.

50 Fritz J, Lindsay W, Matheson J, et al. Is there a subgroup of patients with low back pain likely to benefit from mechanical traction? Results of a randomized clinical trial and subgrouping analysis. Spine 2007;32(26): E793–E800.

51 O'Sullivan P, Beals D. Diagnosis and classification of pelvic girdle pain disorders – Part 1: A mechanism based approach within a biopsychosocial framework. Man Ther 2007;12 (2):86–97.

52 Flynn T, Fritz J, Whitman J, et al. A clinical prediction rule for classifying patients with low back pain who demonstrate short term improvement with spinal manipulation. Spine 2002;27(24):2835–2843.

53 Childs J, Fritz J, Flynn T, et al. A clinical prediction rule to identify patients with low back pain most likely to benefit from spinal manipulation: A validation study. Ann Intern Med 2004;141 (12):920–928.

54 Tseng Y, Wang W, Chen W, et al. Predictors for the immediate responders to cervical manipulation in patients with neck pain. Man Ther 2006;11 (4):306–315.

55 Cleland J, Childs J, Fritz J, et al. Development of a clinical prediction rule for guiding treatment of a subgroup of patients with neck pain: Use of thoracic spine manipulation, exercise, and patient education. Phys Ther 2007;87 (1):9–23.

56 Bombardier C. Outcome assessment in the evaluation of spinal disorders. Summary and general recommendations. Spine 2000;25 (24):3100–3103.

57 Fairbanks J, Davies J, Couper J, et al. The Oswestry Low Back Pain Disability Questionnaire. Physiotherapy 1980;66:271–272.

58 Meade TW, Dyer S, Browne W, et al. Low back pain of mechanical origin: randomized comparison of chiropractic and hospital outpatient treatment. BMJ 1990;300:1431–1437.

59 Hsieh CJ, Phillips RB, Adams AH, et al. Functional outcomes of low back pain: comparison of four treatment groups in a randomized controlled trial. J Manipulative Physiol Ther 1992;15(1):4–9.

60 Roland M, Morris R. A study of the natural history of back pain. Part 1: development of a reliable and sensitive measure of disability in low-back pain. Spine 1983;8:141–144.

61 Fritz JM, Irrgang JJ. A comparison of a modified Oswestry Low Back Pain Disability Questionnaire and the Quebec Back Pain Disability Scale. Phys Ther 2001;81(2):776–788.

62 Walshe D, Radcliffe J. Pain beliefs and perceived physical disability of patients with chronic low back pain. Pain 2002;97:23–31.

63 Vernon H, Mior S. The Neck Disability Index: a study of reliability and validity. J Manipulative Physiol Ther 1991;14(7):409–415.

64 Pinfold M, Niere K, O'Leary E, et al. Validity and internal consistency of a whiplash-specific disability measure. Spine 2004;29(3):263–268.

65 Stratford P, Gill C, Westaway M, et al. Assessing disability and change on individual patients: a report of a patient specific measure. Physiother Can 1995;47:258–263.

66 Westaway M, Stratford P, Binkley J. The patient-specific functional scale: Validation of its use in persons with neck dysfunction. J Orthop Sports Phys Ther 1998;27:331–338.

67 Wolfe F, Smythe HA, Yunnus MB. The American College of Rheumatology 1990: Criteria for classification of fibromyalgia. Arthritis Rheum 1990;33:160–172.

68 Foster N, Pincus T, Underwood M, et al. Understanding the process of care for musculoskeletal conditions – why a biomedical approach is inadequate. Rheumatology 2003;42:401–403.

69 Maher C, Latimer J, Refshauge K. Atlas of clinical tests and measures for low back pain. Melbourne: Australian Physiotherapy Association; 2000.

70 Pincus T, Williams A, Vogel S, et al. The development and testing of the depression, anxiety, and positive outlook scale (DAPOS). Pain 2004;109(1/2):181–188.

71 Orrock P. Profile of members of the Australian Osteopathic Association: Part 1 – The practitioners. Int J Osteopath Med 2009 March; 12(1):14–24.

HVLA thrust techniques

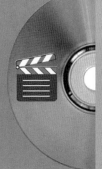

Continued

INTRODUCTION

Part B includes 41 manipulative techniques applied to the spine, thorax & pelvis. All techniques are described using a variable height manipulation couch.

This part of the book relates to specific high-velocity low-amplitude (HVLA) thrust techniques. HVLA thrust techniques are also known by a number of different names, e.g. adjustment, high-velocity thrust, mobilization with impulse, grade V mobilization. Despite the different nomenclature, the common feature in techniques of this type is that they are designed to achieve a joint cavitation (pop or cracking sound). The cause of the popping or cracking sound is open to some speculation.

Information gained from a thorough history, clinical examination and segmental analysis will direct the practitioner towards any possible somatic dysfunction and/or pathology. The use of HVLA thrust techniques is dependent on a diagnosis of somatic dysfunction.

Somatic dysfunction is identified by the S-T-A-R-T of diagnosis:

- S   relates to symptom reproduction
- T   relates to tissue tenderness
- A   relates to asymmetry
- R   relates to range of motion
- T   relates to tissue texture changes

The manual is designed in a format that presents a standardized approach to each region of the spine, thorax & pelvis. If the instructions are followed conscientiously, the novice manipulator will be well placed to achieve a positive outcome from the procedure. The nature of manipulative practice is such that there are many different ways to achieve joint cavitation. Many clinicians achieve extremely high levels of expertise and competence in the use of HVLA thrust techniques. This is the result of many years of individual clinical experience and practice.

This manual is designed to be a safe and effective starting point upon which practitioners can build basic, and then more refined, technical skills. The text lays out the primary and secondary joint leverages required to facilitate effective localization of forces to a specific segment prior to application of the thrust. If the instructions are followed, the resultant thrust is likely to achieve joint gliding and cavitation with the use of minimal force. The joint to be thrust should not be locked, but remain free so that the practitioner can direct a gliding thrust along the joint plane. Appropriate pre-thrust tension is then developed by positioning the joint towards the limit of its available range but not at end range. No text can teach the subtle nuances of HVLA thrust techniques. For example, the sense of appropriate pre-thrust tension is difficult to describe and acquire. Experienced practitioners often use compression as an additional lever. Extensive practice under the supervision of skilled and experienced clinicians is strongly recommended.

The majority of techniques are described using facet apposition locking. In broad terms, facet apposition locking uses combinations of sidebending and rotation. An understanding of the biomechanics associated with coupled movements of the spine in different postures allows the operator to decide on optimal leverages. While rotation and sidebending are the principal leverages used, the more experienced manipulator may include elements of flexion, extension, translation, compression or traction to enhance localization of forces and patient comfort.

Patient relaxation is an essential prerequisite for effective HVLA thrust techniques. This may be facilitated by the use of respiration and other distraction methods.

After making a diagnosis of somatic dysfunction and prior to proceeding with a thrust, it is recommended that the following checklist be used for each of the techniques described in this section:

- Have I excluded all contraindications?
- Have I explained to the patient what I am going to do?
- Do I have informed consent?

- Is the patient well positioned and comfortable?
- Am I in a comfortable and balanced position?
- Do I need to modify any pre-thrust physical or biomechanical factors?

- Have I achieved appropriate pre-thrust tissue tension?
- Am I relaxed and confident to proceed?
- Is the patient relaxed and willing for me to proceed?

8

Cervical and cervicothoracic spine

CERVICAL SPINE HOLDS AND GRIPS

The hold or wrist position selected for any particular technique is that which enables the operator to effectively localize forces to a specific segment of the spine and deliver a high-velocity low-amplitude (HVLA) thrust in a controlled manner. Patient comfort must be a major consideration in selecting the most appropriate hold.

Chin hold

- Operator's left forearm must be over, or slightly in front of, the patient's left ear (Fig. 8.1).
- Operator's fingers lightly clasp the patient's chin (Fig. 8.2).
- Operator's chest should be in contact with the vertex of the patient's head.
- Operator's right hand applies applicator to contact point.

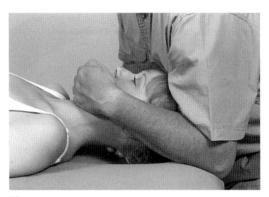

Figure 8.1

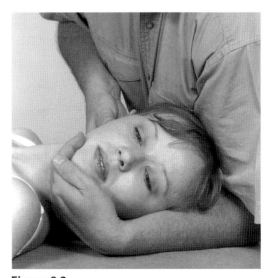

Figure 8.2

Cradle hold

- Patient's left ear resting in the palm of operator's left hand.
- Operator's left hand spread out for maximum contact.
- Operator's right hand applies applicator to contact point and gives support to the patient's occiput.
- The weight of the patient's head and neck is balanced between the operator's left and right hands (Figs 8.3, 8.4).

Wrist position

Operators can select from either the pistol grip (Fig. 8.5) or wrist extension grip (Fig. 8.6).

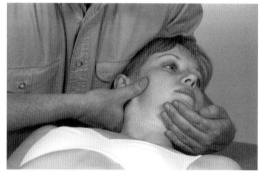

Figure 8.5 Pistol grip Note: radius in line with first metacarpal.

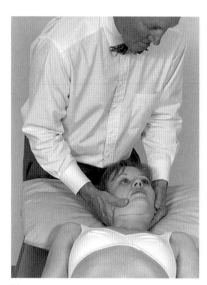

Figure 8.3

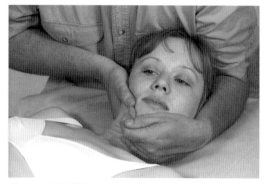

Figure 8.6 Wrist extension grip Note: wrist extension.

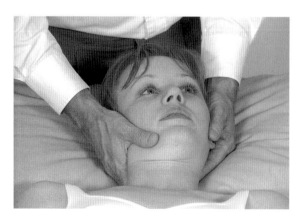

Figure 8.4

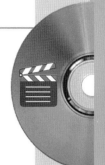

Atlanto-occipital joint C0–C1
Contact point on occiput

Chin hold

Patient supine

Anterior and superior thrust in a curved plane

Assume somatic dysfunction (S-T-A-R-T) is identified and you wish to use a thrust in the plane of the C0–C1 apophysial joint to produce cavitation on the right (Fig. 8.7).

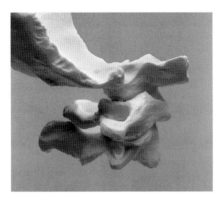

Figure 8.7

KEY

❋ Stabilization

● Applicator

→ Plane of thrust (operator)

⇨ Direction of body movement (patient)

Note: The dimensions for the arrows are not a pictorial representation of the amplitude or force of the thrust.

1. **Contact point**

Right posterior occiput. Medial and posterior to the mastoid process.

2. **Applicator**

Lateral border, proximal or middle phalanx of the operator's right index finger.

3. **Patient positioning**

Supine with the neck in a neutral relaxed position. If necessary, remove pillow or adjust pillow height. The neck should not be in any significant amount of flexion or extension.

4. **Operator stance**

Head of couch, feet spread slightly. Adjust couch height so that the operator can stand as

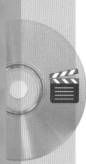

erect as possible and avoid crouching over the patient, as this will limit the technique and restrict delivery of the thrust.

5. Palpation of contact point

Place fingers of both hands gently under the occiput. Lift the head slightly, and gently rotate it to the left, taking the weight of the head in your left hand. Remove your right hand from the occiput and palpate the contact point on the occiput with the tip of your index or middle finger. Ensure that you are medial to, and not on, the mastoid process. Slowly but firmly slide your right index finger, in close approximation to the suboccipital musculature, downward (towards the couch) along the occiput until it approximates the middle or proximal phalanx. Several sliding pressures may be necessary to establish close approximation to the contact point. It is important to obtain a contact point as far along the underside of the occiput as possible and into the suboccipital musculature. This thrust uses a curved plane of movement to produce a cavitation and this positioning ensures that the applicator will not slip during the thrust.

6. Fixation of contact point

Keep your right index finger firmly pressed on the contact point while you flex the other fingers and thumb of the right hand so as to clasp the back of the occiput and head, thereby locking the applicator in position. You must now keep the applicator on the contact point until the technique is complete. Keeping the hands in position, return the head to the neutral position.

7. Chin hold

Keep your right hand in position and slide the left hand, slowly and carefully, forwards until the fingers lightly clasp the chin. Ensure that your left forearm is over or slightly anterior to the ear. Placing the forearm on or behind the ear puts the neck into too much flexion. The head is now controlled by

balancing forces between the right palm and left forearm. Maintain the applicator in position.

8. Vertex contact

Move your body forward slightly so that your chest is in contact with the vertex of the patient's head. The head is now securely cradled between the left forearm, the flexed left elbow, the right palm and your chest. Vertex contact is often useful in a heavy, stiff or difficult case but can, on occasions, be omitted.

9. Positioning for thrust

Step to the right and stand across the right corner of the couch, keeping the hands firmly in position and taking care not to lose pressure on the contact point. Gently introduce a little rotation of the head to the left. Straighten your right wrist so that the radius and first metacarpal are in line. While maintaining firm applicator pressure, allow the right index finger to roll slightly on the contact point as you move your right elbow towards the patient's right shoulder. This facilitates optimal alignment for the thrust, which is in a curved plane because of the shape of the apophysial joint. It is important that your applicator is well beneath the occiput so that you do not slip when applying the thrust along a curved facet plane. Keep your right elbow close to the couch in order to keep the contact point on the occiput (Fig. 8.8).

Add extension and slight sidebending to the right to provide a feeling of tension at the contact point. The extension and right sidebending are introduced by pivoting slightly via the legs and trunk so that your trunk and upper body rotate to the left. Do not attempt to introduce sidebending by moving the hands or arms as this will lead to loss of contact and inaccurate technique. This technique does not use facet apposition locking. The pre-thrust tension is achieved by positioning the occipito-atlantal joint towards the end

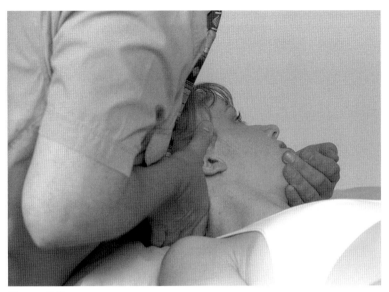

Figure 8.8

range of available joint gliding while avoiding excessive rotation and sidebending leverages. Extensive practice is necessary to develop an appreciation of the required tension.

10. Adjustments to achieve appropriate pre-thrust tension

Ensure the patient remains relaxed. Maintaining all holds, make any necessary minor changes in flexion, extension, sidebending or rotation until you can sense a state of appropriate tension and leverage at the contact point. The patient should not be aware of any pain or discomfort. You should introduce these final adjustments by slight movements of the ankles, knees, hips and trunk, not by altering the position of your hands or arms.

11. Immediately pre-thrust

Relax and adjust your balance as necessary. Keep your head up; looking down impedes the thrust and can cause embarrassing proximity

to the patient. An effective HVLA thrust technique is best achieved if the operator and patient are relaxed and not holding themselves rigid. This is a common impediment to achieving effective cavitation.

Ensure the patient's head and neck remain on the pillow as this facilitates the arrest of the technique and limits excessive amplitude of thrust.

12. Delivering the thrust

This is a difficult technique to master, as the thrust must be applied along a curved plane. Apply a HVLA thrust to the occiput, using both hands, in an anterior and superior direction along a curved plane that follows the shape of the occipito-atlantal articulation (Fig. 8.9).

The thrust, although very rapid, must never be excessively forcible. The aim should be to use the absolute minimum of force necessary to achieve joint cavitation. A common fault arises from the use of excessive amplitude with insufficient velocity of thrust.

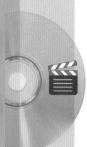

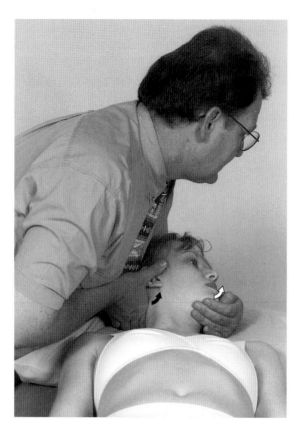

Figure 8.9

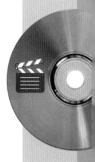

SUMMARY

Atlanto-occipital joint C0–C1 Contact point on occiput

Chin hold

Patient supine

- **Contact point:** Right posterior occiput
- **Applicator:** Lateral border, proximal or middle phalanx
- **Patient positioning:** Supine with the neck in a neutral relaxed position
- **Operator stance:** Head of couch, feet spread slightly
- **Palpation of contact point:** Ensure that you are medial to, and not on, the mastoid process
- **Fixation of contact point**
- **Chin hold:** Ensure your left forearm is over or slightly anterior to the ear
- **Vertex contact:** Optional
- **Positioning for thrust:** Step to the right and stand across the right corner of the couch. Optimal alignment for the thrust is in a curved plane. Keep your right elbow close to the couch in order to keep the contact point on the occiput (Fig. 8.8)
- **Adjustments to achieve appropriate pre-thrust tension**
- **Immediately pre-thrust:** Relax and adjust your balance
- **Delivering the thrust:** The thrust must be applied, using both hands, along a curved plane that follows the shape of the occipito-atlantal articulation (Fig. 8.9)

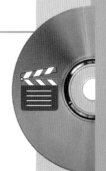

Atlanto-occipital joint C0–C1
Contact point on atlas

Chin hold

Patient supine

Anterior and superior thrust in a curved plane

Assume somatic dysfunction (S-T-A-R-T) is identified and you wish to use a thrust in the plane of the C0–C1 apophysial joint to produce cavitation on the right (Fig. 8.10).

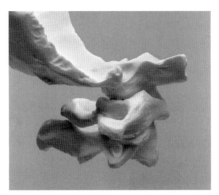

Figure 8.10

KEY

❋ Stabilization

● Applicator

➜ Plane of thrust (operator)

⇨ Direction of body movement (patient)

Note: The dimensions for the arrows are not a pictorial representation of the amplitude or force of the thrust.

1. **Contact point**

Right posterior arch of atlas.

2. **Applicator**

Lateral border, proximal or middle phalanx of operator's right index finger.

3. **Patient positioning**

Supine with the neck in a neutral relaxed position. If necessary, remove pillow or adjust pillow height. The neck should not be in any significant amount of flexion or extension.

4. **Operator stance**

Head of couch, feet spread slightly. Adjust couch height so that the operator can stand as erect as possible and avoid crouching over the

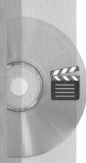

patient as this will limit the technique and restrict delivery of the thrust.

5. Palpation of contact point

Place fingers of both hands gently under the occiput. Lift the head slightly and gently rotate it to the left, taking the weight of the head in your left hand. Remove your right hand from occiput and palpate the contact point on the right posterior arch of the atlas with the tip of your index or middle finger. Slowly but firmly slide your right index finger, in close approximation to the suboccipital musculature, downwards (towards the couch) along the posterior arch of the atlas until it approximates the middle or proximal phalanx. Several sliding pressures may be necessary to establish close approximation to the contact point.

6. Fixation of contact point

Keep your right index finger firmly pressed on the contact point while you flex the other fingers and thumb of the right hand so as to clasp the back of the occiput and head, thereby locking the applicator in position. You must now keep the applicator on the contact point until the technique is complete. Keeping the hands in position, return the head to the neutral position.

7. Chin hold

Keep your right hand in position and slide the left hand, slowly and carefully, forwards until the fingers lightly clasp the chin. Ensure that your left forearm is over or slightly anterior to the ear. Placing the forearm on or behind the ear puts the neck into too much flexion. The head is now controlled by balancing forces between the right palm and left forearm. Maintain the applicator in position.

8. Vertex contact

Move your body forward slightly so that your chest is in contact with the vertex of the patient's head. The head is now securely cradled between the left forearm, the flexed left elbow, the right palm and your chest. Vertex contact is essential in this technique.

9. Positioning for thrust

Step to the right and stand across the right corner of the couch, keeping the hands firmly in position and taking care not to lose pressure on the contact point. Gently introduce a little rotation of the head to the left. Straighten your right wrist so that the radius and first metacarpal are in line. While maintaining firm applicator pressure, allow the right index finger to roll slightly on the contact point as you move your right elbow towards the patient's right shoulder. This facilitates optimal alignment for the thrust, which is in a curved plane because of the shape of the apophysial joint. It is important that your applicator has a firm contact on the atlas so that you do not slip when applying the thrust along a curved facet plane. Keep your right elbow close to the couch in order to keep the contact point on the atlas (Fig. 8.11).

Add extension and slight sidebending to the right to provide a feeling of tension at the contact point. The extension and right sidebending are introduced by pivoting slightly via the legs and trunk so your trunk and upper body rotate to the left. Do not attempt to introduce sidebending by moving the hands or arms, as this will lead to loss of contact and inaccurate technique. This technique does not use facet apposition locking. The pre-thrust tension is achieved by positioning the occipito-atlantal joint towards the end range of available joint gliding while avoiding excessive rotation and sidebending leverages. Extensive practice is necessary to develop an appreciation of the required tension.

10. Adjustments to achieve appropriate pre-thrust tension

Ensure the patient remains relaxed. Maintaining all holds, make any necessary minor changes in flexion, extension, sidebending or rotation until you can sense a state of appropriate tension and leverage at the contact point. The patient should not be aware of any pain or discomfort. You should introduce these final adjustments by slight movements of the ankles, knees, hips and

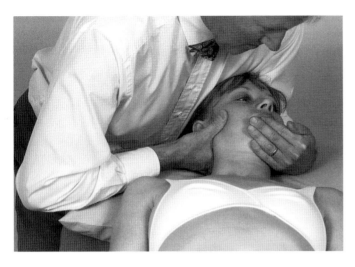

Figure 8.11

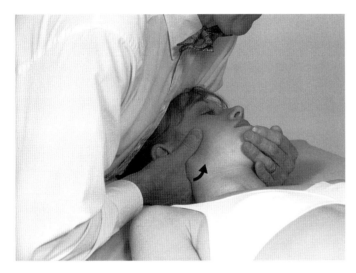

Figure 8.12

trunk, not by altering the position of your hands or arms.

11. Immediately pre-thrust

Relax and adjust your balance as necessary. Keep your head up; looking down impedes the thrust and can cause embarrassing proximity to the patient. An effective HVLA thrust technique is best achieved if the operator and patient are relaxed and not holding themselves rigid. This is a common impediment to achieving effective cavitation.

Ensure the patient's head and neck remain on the pillow as this facilitates the arrest of the technique and limits excessive amplitude of thrust.

12. Delivering the thrust

This is a difficult technique to master, as the thrust must be applied along a curved plane. Apply a HVLA thrust to the posterior arch of the atlas in an anterior and superior direction along a curved plane, which follows the shape of the occipito-atlantal articulation. Apply no simultaneous rapid increase of cervical rotation, extension or sidebending with the left hand (Fig. 8.12).

93

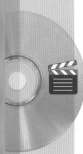

The thrust, although very rapid, must never be excessively forcible. The aim should be to use the absolute minimum force necessary to achieve joint cavitation. A common fault arises from the use of excessive amplitude with insufficient velocity of thrust.

SUMMARY

Atlanto-occipital joint C0–C1 Contact point on atlas

Chin hold

Patient supine

- **Contact point:** Right posterior arch of atlas

- **Applicator:** Lateral border, proximal or middle phalanx

- **Patient positioning:** Supine with the neck in a neutral relaxed position

- **Operator stance:** Head of couch, feet spread slightly

- **Palpation of contact point**

- **Fixation of contact point**

- **Chin hold:** Ensure your left forearm is over or slightly anterior to the ear

- **Vertex contact:** Essential in this technique

- **Positioning for thrust:** Step to the right and stand across the right corner of the couch. Optimal alignment for the thrust is in a curved plane. Keep your right elbow close to the couch in order to keep the contact point on the atlas (Fig. 8.11)

- **Adjustments to achieve appropriate pre-thrust tension**

- **Immediately pre-thrust:** Relax and adjust your balance

- **Delivering the thrust:** The thrust must be applied along a curved plane, which follows the shape of the occipito-atlantal articulation (Fig. 8.12)

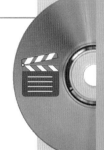

8.3

Atlanto-axial joint C1–2
Chin hold

Patient supine
Rotation thrust

Assume somatic dysfunction (S-T-A-R-T) is identified and you wish to use a thrust in the plane of the atlanto-axial (C1–2) apophysial joint to produce cavitation on the right (Figs 8.13, 8.14).

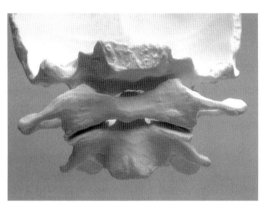

Figure 8.13

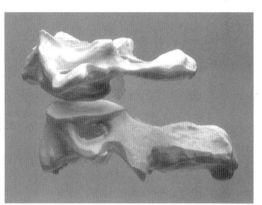

Figure 8.14

KEY

❋ Stabilization

● Applicator

➔ Plane of thrust (operator)

⇨ Direction of body movement (patient)

Note: The dimensions for the arrows are not a pictorial representation of the amplitude or force of the thrust.

1. **Contact point**

Right posterior arch of atlas.

2. **Applicator**

Lateral border, proximal or middle phalanx of operator's right index finger.

3. **Patient positioning**

Supine with the neck in a neutral relaxed position. If necessary, remove pillow or adjust pillow height. The neck should not be in any significant amount of flexion or extension.

4. **Operator stance**

Head of couch, feet spread slightly. Adjust couch height so that the operator can stand as erect as possible and avoid crouching over the

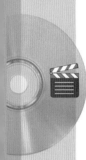

patient as this will limit the technique and restrict delivery of the thrust.

5. **Palpation of contact point**

Place fingers of both hands gently under the occiput. Lift the head slightly and gently rotate it to the left, taking the weight of the head in your left hand. Remove your right hand from the occiput and palpate the region of the right posterior arch of the atlas with the tip of your index or middle finger. Slowly but firmly slide your right index finger downwards (towards the couch) along the posterior arch of the atlas until it approximates the middle or proximal phalanx. Several sliding pressures may be necessary to establish close approximation to the contact point.

6. **Fixation of contact point**

Keep your right index finger firmly pressed upon the contact point while you flex the other fingers and thumb of the right hand, so as to clasp the back of the neck and occiput, thereby locking the applicator in position. You must now keep the applicator on the contact point until the technique is complete. Keeping the hands in position, return the head to the neutral position.

7. **Chin hold**

Keep your right hand in position and slide the left hand, slowly and carefully, forwards until the fingers lightly clasp the chin. Ensure that your left forearm is over, or slightly anterior to, the ear. Placing the forearm on or behind the ear puts the neck into too much flexion. The head is now controlled by balancing forces between the right palm and left forearm. Maintain the applicator in position.

8. **Vertex contact**

Move your body forward slightly so that your chest is in contact with the vertex of the patient's head. The head is now securely cradled between the left forearm, the flexed left elbow, the right palm and your chest. Vertex contact is often useful in a heavy, stiff or difficult case but can, on occasions, be omitted.

9. **Positioning for thrust**

Step to the right and stand across the right corner of the couch, keeping the hands firmly in position and taking care not to lose pressure on the contact point. Gently introduce rotation of the head to the left, to the point at which the posterior arch becomes more obvious under your contact point. Straighten your right wrist so that the radius and first metacarpal are in line. While maintaining firm applicator pressure, allow the right index finger to roll slightly on the contact point as you move your right elbow towards the patient's right shoulder to reach that point when your line of thrust is directed towards the corner of the patient's mouth. The thrust plane is into rotation. Ensure that you maintain a firm contact point on the posterior arch of the atlas and that your applicator is in line with your forearm.

(a) *Primary leverage of rotation.* Maintaining all holds and contact points, complete full rotation of the head and neck to the left until slight tension is palpated in the tissues at your contact point (Fig. 8.15). Maintain firm pressure against the contact point. A common mistake is to use insufficient head and neck rotation.

(b) *Secondary leverage.* This technique uses minimal secondary leverage. This technique does not use facet apposition locking. Extensive practice is necessary to develop an appreciation of the required tension.

10. **Adjustments to achieve appropriate pre-thrust tension**

This is almost a pure rotation thrust but the appropriate tension can be achieved by adjusting flexion, extension and sidebending. The patient should not be aware of any pain or discomfort. Introduce any sidebending, flexion or extension by pivoting slightly via the legs and trunk. Do not attempt to introduce these leverages by moving the hands or arms as this will lead to loss of contact and inaccurate technique.

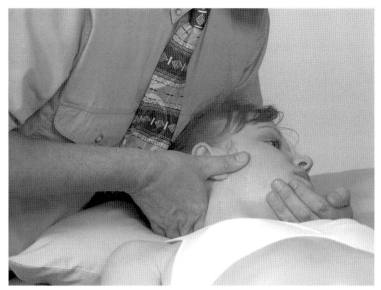

Figure 8.15

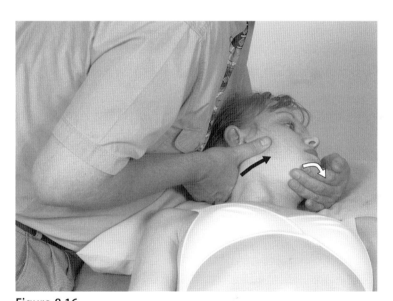

Figure 8.16

11. Immediately pre-thrust

Relax and adjust your balance as necessary. Keep your head up; looking down impedes the thrust and can cause embarrassing proximity to the patient. An effective HVLA thrust technique is best achieved if the operator and patient are relaxed and not holding themselves rigid. This is a common impediment to achieving effective cavitation.

Ensure the patient's head and neck remain on the pillow as this facilitates the arrest of the technique and limits excessive amplitude of thrust.

12. Delivering the thrust

Apply a HVLA thrust to the posterior arch of the atlas directed towards the corner of the patient's mouth. Simultaneously, apply a

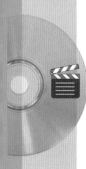

rapid low-amplitude increase of head rotation to the left by supinating the left forearm (Fig. 8.16). This rotation movement of the head is very small but of high velocity. This ensures that the occiput and atlas move as one unit during the thrust. The atlas rotates about the odontoid peg of the axis and cavitation occurs at the right C1–2 articulation. A very rapid contraction of the flexors and adductors of the right shoulder induces the thrust. The thrust, although very rapid, must never be excessively forcible. The aim should be to use the absolute minimum force necessary to achieve joint cavitation. A common fault arises from the use of excessive amplitude with insufficient velocity of thrust.

SUMMARY

Atlanto-axial joint C1–2 Chin hold

Patient supine

Rotation thrust

- **Contact point:** Right posterior arch of atlas

- **Applicator:** Lateral border, proximal or middle phalanx

- **Patient positioning:** Supine with the neck in a neutral relaxed position

- **Operator stance:** Head of couch, feet spread slightly

- **Palpation of contact point**

- **Fixation of contact point**

- **Chin hold:** Ensure your left forearm is over or slightly anterior to the ear

- **Vertex contact:** Optional

- **Positioning for thrust:** Step to the right and stand across the right corner of the couch. Use primary leverage of rotation with minimal secondary leverage. Your direction of thrust is towards the patient's mouth and into rotation (Fig. 8.15)

- **Adjustments to achieve appropriate pre-thrust tension**

- **Immediately pre-thrust:** Relax and adjust your balance

- **Delivering the thrust:** The thrust is directed towards the corner of the patient's mouth. Simultaneously, apply a rapid low-amplitude increase of head rotation to the left. The occiput and atlas move as one unit during the thrust (Fig. 8.16)

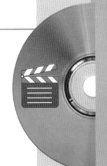

8.4

Atlanto-axial joint C1–2
Cradle hold

Patient supine
Rotation thrust

Assume somatic dysfunction (S-T-A-R-T) is identified and you wish to use a thrust in the plane of the atlanto-axial (C1–2) apophysial joint to produce cavitation on the right (Figs 8.17, 8.18).

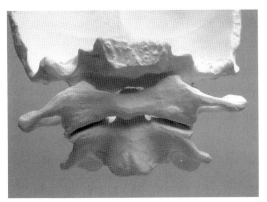

Figure 8.17

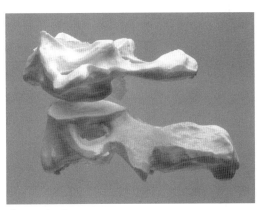

Figure 8.18

KEY

 Stabilization

● Applicator

➜ Plane of thrust (operator)

⇨ Direction of body movement (patient)

Note: The dimensions for the arrows are not a pictorial representation of the amplitude or force of the thrust.

1. Contact point

Right posterior arch of atlas.

2. Applicator

Lateral border, proximal or middle phalanx of operator's right index finger.

3. Patient positioning

Supine with the neck in a neutral relaxed position. If necessary, remove pillow or adjust pillow height. The neck should not be in any significant amount of flexion or extension.

4. Operator stance

Head of couch, feet spread slightly. Adjust couch height so that the operator can stand as erect as possible and avoid crouching over the

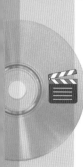

patient as this will limit the technique and restrict delivery of the thrust.

5. Palpation of contact point

Place fingers of both hands gently under the occiput. Lift the head slightly and gently rotate it to the left, taking the weight of the head in your left hand. Remove your right hand from the occiput and palpate the region of the right posterior arch of the atlas with the tip of your index or middle finger. Slowly but firmly slide your right index finger downwards (towards the couch) along the posterior arch of the atlas until it approximates the middle or proximal phalanx. Several sliding pressures may be necessary to establish close approximation to the contact point.

6. Fixation of contact point

Keep your right index finger firmly pressed upon the contact point while you flex the other fingers and thumb of the right hand so as to clasp the back of the neck and occiput, thereby locking the applicator in position. You must now keep the applicator on the contact point until the technique is complete. Keeping the hands in position, return the head to the neutral position.

7. Cradle hold

Keep your left hand under the head and spread the fingers out for maximum contact. Keep the patient's ear resting in the palm of your left hand. Flex the left wrist, allowing you to cradle the patient's head in your palm, flexed wrist and anterior aspect of forearm. Keep your right index finger firmly on the contact point and press the right palm against the occiput. The weight of the patient's head and neck is now balanced between your left and right hands with the cervical positioning controlled by the converging pressures of your two hands and arms.

8. Vertex contact

None in this technique.

9. Positioning for thrust

The elbows are held close to or only slightly away from your sides. This is an essential feature of the cradle hold method. Stand easily upright at the head of the couch and do not step to the right as in the chin hold method.

(a) *Primary leverage of rotation.* Maintaining all holds and contact points, complete the rotation of the head and neck to the left until tension is palpated at the contact point. Supination of the left wrist and forearm and simultaneous pronation of the right wrist and forearm achieve the rotation movement (Fig. 8.19). Do not lose firm pressure on the contact point. Do not force rotation; take it up fully but carefully. A common mistake is to use insufficient primary leverage of head and neck rotation.

(b) *Secondary leverage.* This technique uses minimal secondary leverage. This technique does not use facet apposition locking. Extensive practice is necessary to develop an appreciation of the required tension.

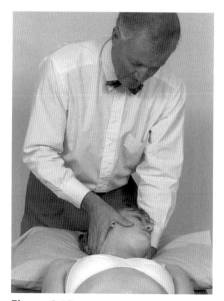

Figure 8.19

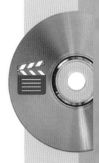

10. Adjustments to achieve appropriate pre-thrust tension

This is almost a pure rotation thrust, but the appropriate tension can be achieved by adjusting flexion, extension and sidebending. The patient should not be aware of any pain or discomfort. The operator makes final minor adjustments by introducing any sidebending, flexion or extension with slight movements of the wrists, arms and shoulders.

11. Immediately pre-thrust

Relax and adjust your balance as necessary. Keep your head up; looking down impedes the thrust and can cause embarrassing proximity to the patient. An effective HVLA thrust technique is best achieved if the operator and patient are relaxed and not holding themselves rigid. This is a common impediment to achieving effective cavitation.

Ensure the patient's head and neck remain on the pillow as this facilitates the arrest of the technique and limits excessive amplitude of thrust.

12. Delivering the thrust

Apply a HVLA thrust to the posterior arch of the atlas directed towards the corner of the patient's mouth. This thrust is generated by rapid pronation of your right forearm. Simultaneously, apply a rapid low-amplitude increase of head rotation to the left by supinating the left forearm (Fig. 8.20). This rotation movement of the head is very small but of high velocity. This ensures that the occiput and atlas move as one unit during the thrust. The atlas rotates about the odontoid peg of the axis and cavitation occurs at the right C1–2 articulation. This is a HVLA 'flick' type thrust. Coordination between the left and right hands and forearms is critical.

The thrust, although very rapid, must never be excessively forcible. The aim should be to use the absolute minimum force necessary to achieve joint cavitation. A common fault arises from the use of excessive amplitude with insufficient velocity of thrust.

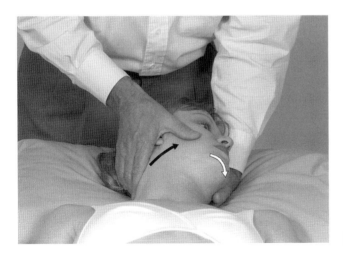

Figure 8.20

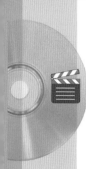

SUMMARY

Atlanto-axial joint C1–2 Cradle hold

Patient supine

Rotation thrust

- **Contact point:** Right posterior arch of atlas
- **Applicator:** Lateral border, proximal or middle phalanx
- **Patient positioning:** Supine with the neck in a neutral relaxed position
- **Operator stance:** Head of couch, feet spread slightly
- **Palpation of contact point**
- **Fixation of contact point**
- **Cradle hold:** The weight of the patient's head and neck is balanced between your left and right hands with cervical positioning controlled by the converging pressures
- **Vertex contact:** None
- **Positioning for thrust:** Stand upright at the head of the couch. The elbows are held close to or only slightly away from your sides. Use primary leverage of rotation with minimal secondary leverage. Your direction of thrust is towards the patient's mouth and into rotation (Fig. 8.19)
- **Adjustments to achieve appropriate pre-thrust tension**
- **Immediately pre-thrust:** Relax and adjust your balance
- **Delivering the thrust:** The thrust is directed towards the corner of the patient's mouth. Simultaneously, apply a rapid low-amplitude increase of head rotation to the left. The occiput and atlas move as one unit during the thrust (Fig. 8.20)

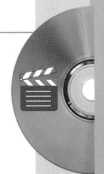

Cervical spine C2–7
Up-slope gliding

Chin hold
Patient supine

Assume somatic dysfunction (S-T-A-R-T) is identified and you wish to use an upwards and forwards gliding thrust, parallel to the apophysial joint plane, to produce cavitation at C4–5 on the right (Figs 8.21, 8.22).

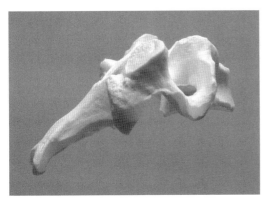

Figure 8.21

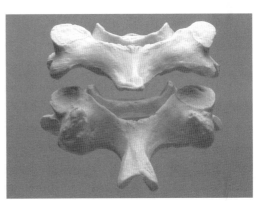

Figure 8.22

KEY

❋ Stabilization

● Applicator

→ Plane of thrust (operator)

⇨ Direction of body movement (patient)

Note: The dimensions for the arrows are not a pictorial representation of the amplitude or force of the thrust.

1. **Contact point**

Posterolateral aspect of right C4 articular pillar.

2. **Applicator**

Lateral border, proximal or middle phalanx of operator's right index finger.

3. **Patient positioning**

Supine with the neck in a neutral relaxed position. If necessary, remove pillow or adjust pillow height. The neck should not be in any significant amount of flexion or extension.

4. **Operator stance**

Head of couch, feet spread slightly. Adjust couch height so that you can stand as erect as

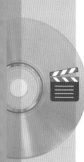

possible and avoid crouching over the patient as this will limit the technique and restrict delivery of the thrust.

5. Palpation of contact point

Place fingers of both hands gently under the occiput. Rotate the head to the left, taking its weight in your left hand. Remove your right hand from the occiput and palpate the right articular pillar of C4 with the tip of your index or middle finger. Slowly but firmly slide your right index finger downwards (towards the couch) along the articular pillar until it approximates the middle or proximal phalanx. Several sliding pressures may be necessary to establish close approximation to the contact point.

6. Fixation of contact point

Keep your right index finger firmly pressed upon the contact point while you flex the other fingers and thumb of the right hand so as to clasp the back of the neck and thereby lock the applicator in position. You must now keep the applicator on the contact point until the technique is complete. Keeping the hands in position, return the head to the neutral position.

7. Chin hold

Keeping your right hand in position, slide the left hand slowly and carefully forwards until the fingers lightly clasp the chin. Ensure that your left forearm is over or slightly anterior to the ear. Placing the forearm on or behind the ear puts the neck into too much flexion. The head is now controlled by balancing forces between the right palm and left forearm. Maintain the applicator in position.

8. Vertex contact

Move your body forward slightly so that your chest is in contact with the vertex of the patient's head. The head is now securely cradled between your left forearm, the flexed left elbow, the right palm and your chest. Vertex contact is often useful in a heavy, stiff or difficult case but can, on occasions, be omitted.

9. Positioning for thrust

Step to the right and stand across the right corner of the couch, keeping the hands firmly in position and taking care not to lose pressure on the contact point. Straighten the right wrist so that the radius and first metacarpal are in line. Maintaining applicator pressure, allow the right index finger to roll slightly on the contact point to align your right wrist and forearm with the thrust plane, which is upwards and towards the midline in the direction of the patient's left eye. Keep the right elbow close to the couch in order to maintain the contact point on the posterolateral aspect of the articular pillar.

(a) *Primary leverage of rotation.* Maintaining all holds and contact points, complete the rotation of the head and neck to the left until tension is palpated at the contact point (Fig. 8.23). Do not lose firm pressure at the contact point. A common mistake is to use insufficient primary leverage of head and neck rotation.

(b) *Secondary leverage.* Add a very small degree of sidebending to the right, down to and including the C3–4 segment but leaving C4–5 free to move. The operator pivoting slightly, via the legs and trunk, introduces the right sidebending, so that the trunk and upper body rotate to the left, enabling the hands and arms to remain in position (Fig. 8.24). Do not attempt to introduce sidebending by moving the hands or arms as this will lead to loss of contact and inaccurate technique.

10. Adjustments to achieve appropriate pre-thrust tension

Ensure your patient remains relaxed. Maintaining all holds, make any necessary changes in flexion, extension, sidebending or rotation until you can sense a state of appropriate tension and leverage. The patient should not be aware of any pain or discomfort. You make these final adjustments by slight movements of your ankles, knees, hips and trunk, not by altering the position of the hands or arms.

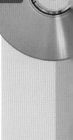

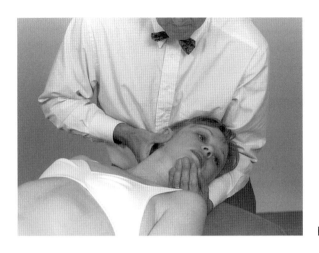

Figure 8.23

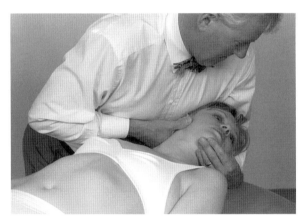

Figure 8.24

11. Immediately pre-thrust

Relax and adjust your balance as necessary. Keep your head up; looking down impedes the thrust and can cause embarrassing proximity to the patient. An effective HVLA thrust technique is best achieved if both the operator and patient are relaxed and not holding themselves rigid. This is a common impediment to achieving effective cavitation.

Ensure the patient's head and neck remain on the pillow as this facilitates the arrest of the technique and limits excessive amplitude of thrust.

12. Delivering the thrust

Apply a HVLA thrust to the right articular pillar of C4. The thrust is upwards and towards the midline in the direction of the patient's left eye, parallel to the apophysial joint plane.

Simultaneously, apply a slight, rapid increase of rotation of the head and neck to the left but do not increase the sidebending leverage (Fig. 8.25). The increase of rotation to the left is accomplished by slight supination of the left wrist and forearm. The thrust is induced by

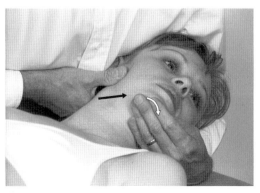

Figure 8.25

105

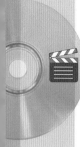

a very rapid contraction of the flexors and adductors of the right shoulder and, if necessary, trunk and lower limb movement.

The thrust, although very rapid, must never be excessively forcible. The aim should be to use the absolute minimum force necessary to achieve joint cavitation. A common fault arises from the use of excessive amplitude with insufficient velocity of thrust.

SUMMARY

Cervical spine C2–7 Up-slope gliding

Chin hold

Patient supine

- **Contact point:** Posterolateral aspect of right C4 articular pillar

- **Applicator:** Lateral border, proximal or middle phalanx

- **Patient positioning:** Supine with the neck in a neutral relaxed position

- **Operator stance:** Head of couch, feet spread slightly

- **Palpation of contact point**

- **Fixation of contact point**

- **Chin hold:** Ensure your left forearm is over or slightly anterior to the ear

- **Vertex contact:** Optional

- **Positioning for thrust:** Step to the right and stand across the right corner of the couch. Introduce primary leverage of rotation left (Fig. 8.23) and a small degree of secondary leverage of sidebending right. Keep the right elbow close to the couch in order to maintain the contact point on the posterolateral aspect of the C4 articular pillar (Fig. 8.24)

- **Adjustments to achieve appropriate pre-thrust tension**

- **Immediately pre-thrust:** Relax and adjust your balance

- **Delivering the thrust:** The thrust is directed towards the patient's left eye. Simultaneously, apply a slight, rapid increase of rotation of the head and neck to the left with no increase of sidebending to the right (Fig. 8.25)

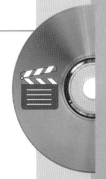

Cervical spine C2–7
Up-slope gliding

Chin hold
Patient supine – variation

Assume somatic dysfunction (S-T-A-R-T) is identified and you wish to use an upward and forward gliding thrust, parallel to the apophysial joint plane, to produce cavitation at C4–5 on the right (Figs 8.26, 8.27).

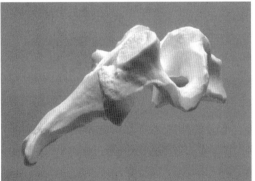

Figure 8.26

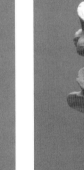

Figure 8.27

KEY

✳ Stabilization

● Applicator

→ Plane of thrust (operator)

⇨ Direction of body movement
(patient)

Note: The dimensions for the arrows are not a pictorial representation of the amplitude or force of the thrust.

1. **Contact point**

Posterolateral aspect of right C4 articular pillar.

2. **Applicator**

Lateral border, proximal or middle phalanx of operator's right index finger.

3. **Patient positioning**

Supine with the neck in a neutral relaxed position. If necessary, remove pillow or adjust pillow height. The neck should not be in any significant amount of flexion or extension.

4. **Operator stance**

Head of couch, feet spread slightly. Adjust couch height so that you can stand as erect as possible and avoid crouching over the patient as this will limit the technique and restrict delivery of the thrust.

5. Palpation of contact point

Place fingers of both hands gently under the occiput. Rotate the head to the left, taking its weight in your left hand. Remove your right hand from the occiput and palpate the right articular pillar of C4 with the tip of your index or middle finger. Slowly but firmly slide your right index finger downwards (towards the couch) along the articular pillar until it approximates the middle or proximal phalanx. Several sliding pressures may be necessary to establish close approximation to the contact point.

6. Fixation of contact point

Keep your right index finger firmly pressed upon the contact point while you flex the other fingers and thumb of the right hand so as to clasp the back of the neck and thereby lock the applicator in position. You must now keep the applicator on the contact point until the technique is complete. Keeping the hands in position, return the head to the neutral position.

7. Chin hold

Step to the right while allowing your applicator to roll on the contact point. Keeping your right hand in position, slide the left hand slowly and carefully forwards until the fingers lightly clasp the chin (Fig. 8.28). Ensure that your left forearm is over or slightly

anterior to the ear. Placing the forearm on or behind the ear puts the neck into too much flexion. The head is now controlled by balancing forces between the right palm and left forearm. Maintain the applicator in position.

8. Vertex contact

Move your body forward slightly so that your chest is in contact with the vertex of the patient's head. The head is now securely cradled between your left forearm, the flexed left elbow, the right palm and your chest. Vertex contact is often useful in a heavy, stiff or difficult case but can, on occasions, be omitted.

9. Positioning for thrust

Keeping the hands firmly in position and taking care not to lose pressure on the contact point, straighten the right wrist so that the radius and first metacarpal are in line. Maintaining applicator pressure, allow the right index finger to roll slightly on the contact point to align your right wrist and forearm with the thrust plane, which is upwards and towards the midline in the direction of the patient's left eye. Keep the right elbow close to the couch in order to maintain the contact point on the posterolateral aspect of the articular pillar.

(a) *Primary leverage of rotation.* Maintaining all holds and contact points, complete the rotation of the head and neck to the left until tension is palpated at the contact point (Fig. 8.29). Do not lose firm

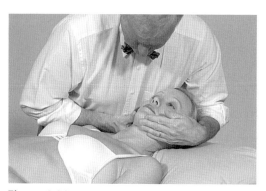
Figure 8.28

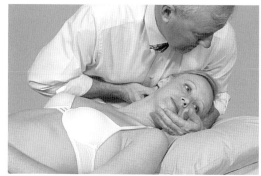
Figure 8.29

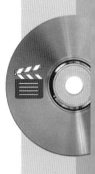

pressure at the contact point. A common mistake is to use insufficient primary leverage of head and neck rotation.

(b) *Secondary leverage.* Add a very small degree of sidebending to the right, down to and including the C3–4 segment but leaving C4–5 free to move. The operator pivoting slightly, via the legs and trunk, introduces the right sidebending, so that the trunk and upper body rotate to the left, enabling the hands and arms to remain in position (Fig. 8.30). Do not attempt to introduce sidebending by moving the hands or arms as this will lead to loss of contact and inaccurate technique.

10. Adjustments to achieve appropriate pre-thrust tension

Ensure your patient remains relaxed. Maintaining all holds, make any necessary changes in flexion, extension, sidebending or rotation until you can sense a state of appropriate tension and leverage. The patient should not be aware of any pain or discomfort. You make these final adjustments by slight movements of your ankles, knees, hips and trunk, not by altering the position of the hands or arms.

11. Immediately pre-thrust

Relax and adjust your balance as necessary. Keep your head up; looking down impedes the thrust and can cause embarrassing proximity to the patient. An effective HVLA thrust technique is best achieved if both the operator and patient are relaxed and not holding themselves rigid. This is a common impediment to achieving effective cavitation.

Ensure the patient's head and neck remain on the pillow as this facilitates the arrest of the technique and limits excessive amplitude of thrust.

12. Delivering the thrust

Apply a HVLA thrust to the right articular pillar of C4. The thrust is upwards and towards the midline in the direction of the patient's left eye, parallel to the apophysial joint plane. Simultaneously, apply a slight, rapid increase of rotation of the head and neck to the left but do not increase the sidebending leverage (Fig. 8.31). The increase of rotation to the left is accomplished by slight supination of the left wrist and forearm. The thrust is induced by a very rapid contraction of the flexors and adductors of the right shoulder and, if necessary, trunk and lower limb movement.

The thrust, although very rapid, must never be excessively forcible. The aim should be to use the absolute minimum force necessary to achieve joint cavitation. A common fault arises from the use of excessive amplitude with insufficient velocity of thrust.

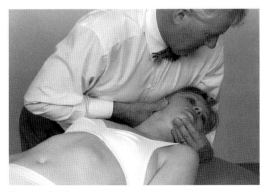

Figure 8.30

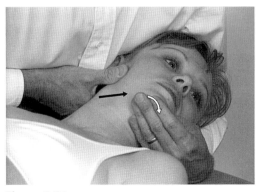

Figure 8.31

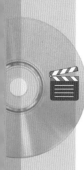

SUMMARY

Cervical spine C2–7 Up-slope gliding

Chin hold

Patient supine

- **Contact point:** Posterolateral aspect of right C4 articular pillar

- **Applicator:** Lateral border, proximal or middle phalanx

- **Patient positioning:** Supine with the neck in a neutral relaxed position

- **Operator stance:** Head of couch, feet spread slightly

- **Palpation of contact point**

- **Fixation of contact point**

- **Chin hold:** Step to the right before taking up chin hold (Fig. 8.28). Take up chin hold and ensure your left forearm is over or slightly anterior to the ear

- **Vertex contact:** Optional

- **Positioning for thrust:** Introduce primary leverage of rotation left (Fig. 8.29) and a small degree of secondary leverage of sidebending right. Keep the right elbow close to the couch in order to maintain the contact point on the posterolateral aspect of the C4 articular pillar (Fig. 8.30)

- **Adjustments to achieve appropriate pre-thrust tension**

- **Immediately pre-thrust:** Relax and adjust your balance

- **Delivering the thrust:** The thrust is directed towards the patient's left eye. Simultaneously, apply a slight, rapid increase of rotation of the head and neck to the left with no increase of sidebending to the right (Fig. 8.31)

8.7

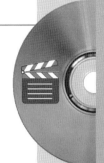

Cervical spine C2–7
Up-slope gliding

Cradle hold
Patient supine

Assume somatic dysfunction (S-T-A-R-T) is identified and you wish to use an upward and forward gliding thrust, parallel to the apophysial joint plane, to produce cavitation at C4–5 on the right (Figs 8.32, 8.33).

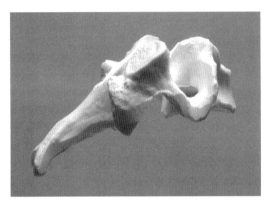

Figure 8.32

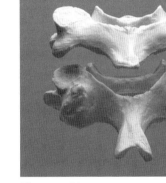

Figure 8.33

KEY

✳ Stabilization

● Applicator

➔ Plane of thrust (operator)

⇨ Direction of body movement (patient)

Note: The dimensions for the arrows are not a pictorial representation of the amplitude or force of the thrust.

1. **Contact point**

Posterolateral aspect of the right articular pillar of C4.

2. **Applicator**

Lateral border, proximal or middle phalanx of operator's right index finger.

3. **Patient positioning**

Supine with the neck in a neutral relaxed position. If necessary, remove or adjust pillow height. The technique should not normally be executed in any significant degree of flexion or extension.

4. **Operator stance**

Head of couch, feet spread slightly. Adjust couch height so that you can stand as erect as

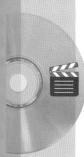

possible and avoid crouching over the patient as this will limit the technique and restrict delivery of the thrust.

5. Palpation of contact point

Place fingers of both hands gently under the occiput. Lift the head to throw the articular pillars into prominence. Rotate the head slightly to the left, taking its weight in your left hand. Remove your right hand from the occiput and palpate the right articular pillar of C4 with the tip of your right index finger. Slowly but firmly slide your right forefinger downwards (towards the couch) along the articular pillar until it approximates the middle or proximal phalanx. Several sliding pressures may be necessary to establish close approximation to the contact point.

6. Fixation of contact point

Keep your right index finger firmly pressed upon the contact point while you flex the other fingers and thumb of the right hand so as to clasp the back of the neck and thereby lock the applicator in position. You must now keep the applicator on the contact point until the technique is complete. Keeping the hands in position, return the head to the neutral position.

7. Cradle hold

Keep your left hand under the head and spread the fingers out for maximum contact. Keep the patient's ear resting in the palm of the your left hand. Flex the left wrist, allowing you to cradle the patient's head in your palm, flexed wrist and anterior aspect of forearm. Keep your right index finger firmly on the contact point and press the right palm against the occiput. The weight of the patient's head and neck is now balanced between your left and right hands with the cervical positioning controlled by the converging pressures of your two hands and arms. When treating the lower cervical segments, the middle or distal phalanx may be used as the applicator.

8. Vertex contact

None in this technique.

9. Positioning for thrust

The elbows are held close to or only slightly away from your sides. This is an essential feature of the cradle hold method. Stand easily upright at the head of the couch and do not step to the right as in the chin hold method.

(a) *Primary leverage of rotation.* Maintaining all holds and contact points, complete the rotation of the head and neck to the left until tension is palpated at the contact point. Supination of the left wrist and forearm and simultaneous pronation of the right wrist and forearm achieve the rotation movement (Fig. 8.34). Do not lose firm pressure on the contact point. Do not force rotation; take it up fully but carefully. A common mistake is to use insufficient primary leverage of head and neck rotation.

(b) *Secondary leverage.* Add a very small degree of sidebending to the right, down to and including the C3–4 segment but leaving C4–5 free to move. This is achieved by moving the right arm a little forward and the left arm a little back or by rotating the trunk and upper body to the left (Fig. 8.35). *Note:* strong sidebending will lock the neck.

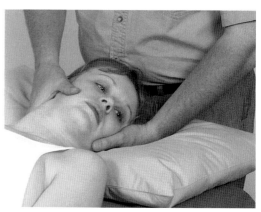

Figure 8.34

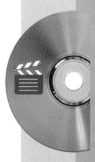

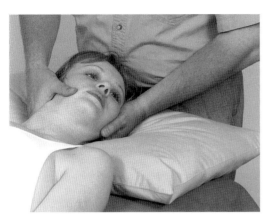

Figure 8.35

10. **Adjustments to achieve appropriate pre-thrust tension**

Ensure your patient remains relaxed. Maintaining all holds, make any necessary changes in flexion, extension, sidebending or rotation until you can sense a state of appropriate tension and leverage. The patient should not be aware of any pain or discomfort. You make these final adjustments by slight movements of your ankles, knees, hips and trunk, not by altering the position of the hands or arms.

11. **Immediately pre-thrust**

Relax and adjust your balance as necessary. Keep your head up; looking down impedes the thrust and can cause embarrassing proximity to the patient. An effective HVLA thrust technique is best achieved if both the operator and patient are relaxed and not holding themselves rigid. This is a common impediment to achieving effective cavitation.

Ensure the patient's head and neck remain on the pillow as this facilitates the arrest of the

technique and limits excessive amplitude of thrust.

12. **Delivering the thrust**

Apply a HVLA thrust to the right articular pillar of C4. The thrust is upwards and towards the midline in the direction of the patient's left eye, parallel to the apophysial joint plane (Fig. 8.36). This thrust is generated by rapid pronation of your right forearm. Simultaneously, apply a slight rapid increase of rotation of the head and neck to the left, but do not increase sidebending leverages. The increase of rotation to the left is accomplished by slight supination of the left wrist and forearm and is coordinated to match the thrust upon the contact point. This is a HVLA 'flick' type thrust. Coordination between the left and right hands and forearms is critical.

The thrust, although very rapid, must never be excessively forcible. The aim should be to use the absolute minimum force necessary to achieve joint cavitation. A common fault arises from the use of excessive amplitude with insufficient velocity of thrust.

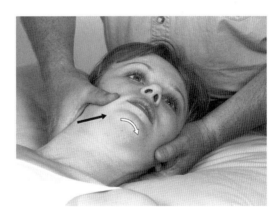

Figure 8.36

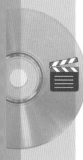

SUMMARY

Cervical spine C2–7 Up-slope gliding

Cradle hold

Patient supine

- **Contact point:** Posterolateral aspect of the right C4 articular pillar
- **Applicator:** Lateral border, proximal or middle phalanx
- **Patient positioning:** Supine with the neck in a neutral relaxed position
- **Operator stance:** Head of couch, feet spread slightly
- **Palpation of contact point**
- **Fixation of contact point**
- **Cradle hold:** The weight of the patient's head and neck is balanced between your left and right hands with cervical positioning controlled by the converging pressures
- **Vertex contact:** None
- **Positioning for thrust:** Stand upright at the head of the couch. The elbows are held close to or only slightly away from your sides. Introduce primary leverage of rotation to the left (Fig. 8.34) and a small degree of secondary leverage of sidebending right (Fig. 8.35). Maintain the contact point on the posterolateral aspect of the C4 articular pillar
- **Adjustments to achieve appropriate pre-thrust tension**
- **Immediately pre-thrust:** Relax and adjust your balance
- **Delivering the thrust:** The thrust is directed towards the patient's left eye. Simultaneously, apply a slight, rapid increase of rotation of the head and neck to the left with no increase of sidebending to the right (Fig. 8.36)

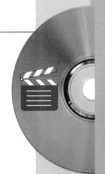

8.8

Cervical spine C2–7
Up-slope gliding

Cradle hold
Patient supine
Reversed primary and secondary leverage

In certain circumstances, the operator might wish to perform an up-slope gliding thrust but minimize the extent of head and neck rotation. Assume somatic dysfunction (S-T-A-R-T) is identified and you wish to use an upward and forward gliding thrust, parallel to the apophysial joint plane, to produce cavitation at C4–5 on the right (Figs 8.37, 8.38).

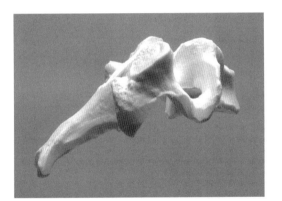

Figure 8.37

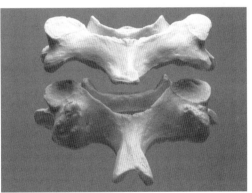

Figure 8.38

KEY

❋ Stabilization

● Applicator

➔ Plane of thrust (operator)

⇨ Direction of body movement (patient)

Note: The dimensions for the arrows are not a pictorial representation of the amplitude or force of the thrust.

---

1. **Contact point**

Posterolateral aspect of the right articular pillar of C4.

2. **Applicator**

Lateral border, proximal or middle phalanx of operator's right index finger.

3. **Patient positioning**

Supine with the neck in a neutral relaxed position. If necessary, remove or adjust pillow height. The technique should not normally be executed in any significant degree of flexion or extension.

4. **Operator stance**

Head of couch, feet spread slightly. Adjust couch height so that you can stand as erect as

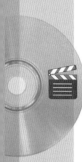

possible and avoid crouching over the patient as this will limit the technique and restrict delivery of the thrust.

5. Palpation of contact point

Place fingers of both hands gently under the occiput. Lift the head to throw the articular pillars into prominence. Rotate the head slightly to the left, taking its weight in your left hand. Remove your right hand from the occiput and palpate the right articular pillar of C4 with the tip of your right index finger. Slowly but firmly slide your right forefinger downwards (towards the couch) along the articular pillar until it approximates the middle or proximal phalanx. Several sliding pressures may be necessary to establish close approximation to the contact point.

6. Fixation of contact point

Keep your right index finger firmly pressed upon the contact point while you flex the other fingers and thumb of the right hand so as to clasp the back of the neck and thereby lock the applicator in position. You must now keep the applicator on the contact point until the technique is complete. Keeping the hands in position, return the head to the neutral position.

7. Cradle hold

Keep your left hand under the head and spread the fingers out for maximum contact. Keep the patient's ear resting in the palm of the your left hand. Flex the left wrist, allowing you to cradle the patient's head in your palm, flexed wrist and anterior aspect of forearm. Keep your right index finger firmly on the contact point and press the right palm against the occiput. The weight of the patient's head and neck is now balanced between your left and right hands, with the cervical positioning controlled by the converging pressures of your two hands and arms. When treating the lower cervical segments, the middle or distal phalanx may be used as the applicator.

8. Vertex contact

None in this technique.

9. Positioning for thrust

The intent with this technique is to perform an up-slope gliding thrust but to limit the amount of head and neck rotation. This modification requires a greater emphasis upon the use of sidebending to achieve joint locking. It is critical that the direction of thrust be parallel to the apophysial joint plane in an up-slope direction. There should be no exaggeration of the sidebending leverage.

The elbows are held close to or only slightly away from your sides. This is an essential feature of the cradle hold method. Stand easily upright at the head of the couch and do not step to the right as in the chin hold method.

(a) *Primary leverage of sidebending.*
   Maintaining all holds and contact points, gently introduce sidebending of the head and neck to the right until tension is palpated at the contact point (Fig. 8.39). To introduce the right sidebending, the operator pivots slightly

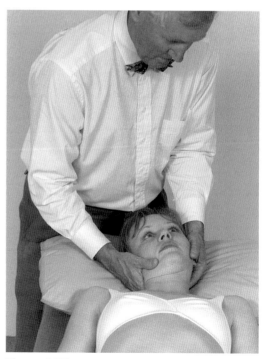

Figure 8.39

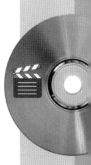

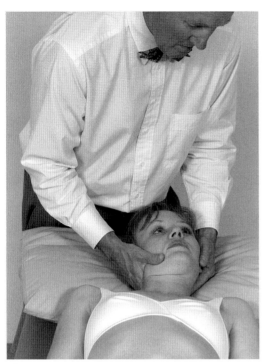

Figure 8.40

discomfort. You make these final adjustments by slight movements of your ankles, knees, hips and trunk, not by altering the position of the hands or arms.

11. Immediately pre-thrust

Relax and adjust your balance as necessary. Keep your head up; looking down impedes the thrust and can cause embarrassing proximity to the patient. An effective HVLA thrust technique is best achieved if both the operator and patient are relaxed and not holding themselves rigid. This is a common impediment to achieving effective cavitation.

Ensure the patient's head and neck remain on the pillow as this facilitates the arrest of the technique and limits excessive amplitude of thrust.

12. Delivering the thrust

Apply a HVLA thrust to the right articular pillar of C4. The thrust is upwards and towards the midline in the direction of the patient's left eye, parallel to the apophysial joint plane (Fig. 8.41). This thrust is generated by rapid pronation of your right forearm. Simultaneously, apply a slight rapid increase of rotation of the head and neck to the left. A key element in this technique is to avoid exaggeration of the primary leverage of sidebending when the thrust is applied. The increase of rotation to the left is accomplished by slight supination of left wrist and forearm and coordinated to match the thrust upon the contact point. This is a HVLA 'flick' type thrust. Coordination between the left and right hands and forearms is critical.

It must be appreciated that the use of sidebending as a primary leverage is predicated upon the operator's desire to limit the amount of head and neck rotation. Generally, when sidebending is used as a primary leverage, the aim will be to thrust in a down-slope direction. Exaggeration of the sidebending leverage in this technique must be avoided. Sidebending enhances locking but does not assist with an up-slope gliding thrust. The thrust in this technique is accompanied by

via the legs and trunk so that the trunk and upper body rotate to the left, enabling the hands and arms to remain in position. Do not lose firm contact with your contact point on the articular pillar of C4. A common mistake is to use insufficient primary leverage of head and neck sidebending.

(b) *Secondary leverage.* Add a little rotation to the left, down to and including the C3–4 segment but leaving C4–5 free to move (Fig. 8.40). This requires extensive practice before one develops a refined 'tension sense'. Movement of your hands and forearms introduces the rotation.

10. Adjustments to achieve appropriate pre-thrust tension

Ensure your patient remains relaxed. Maintaining all holds, make any necessary changes in flexion, extension, sidebending or rotation until you can sense a state of appropriate tension and leverage. The patient should not be aware of any pain or

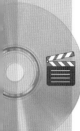

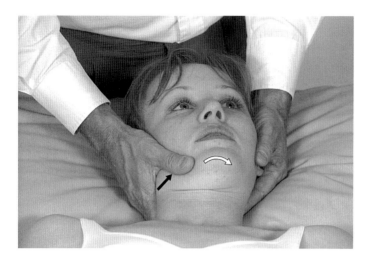

Figure 8.41

slight exaggeration of the secondary leverage of rotation and is directed towards the patient's opposite eye.

The thrust, although very rapid, must never be excessively forcible. The aim

should be to use the absolute minimum force necessary to achieve joint cavitation. A common fault arises from the use of excessive amplitude with insufficient velocity of thrust.

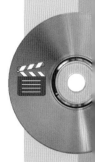

SUMMARY

Cervical spine C2–7 Up-slope gliding

Cradle hold

Patient supine

Reversed primary and secondary leverage

- **Contact point:** Posterolateral aspect of the right C4 articular pillar

- **Applicator:** Lateral border, proximal or middle phalanx

- **Patient positioning:** Supine with the neck in a neutral relaxed position

- **Operator stance:** Head of couch, feet spread slightly

- **Palpation of contact point**

- **Fixation of contact point**

- **Cradle hold:** The weight of the patient's head and neck is now balanced between your left and right hands with cervical positioning controlled by the converging pressures

- **Vertex contact:** None

- **Positioning for thrust:** Stand upright at the head of the couch. The elbows are held close to or only slightly away from your sides. Introduce primary leverage of sidebending to the right (Fig. 8.39) and a small degree of secondary leverage of rotation left (Fig. 8.40). Maintain the contact point on the posterolateral aspect of the C4 articular pillar

- **Adjustments to achieve appropriate pre-thrust tension**

- **Immediately pre-thrust:** Relax and adjust your balance

- **Delivering the thrust:** The thrust is directed towards the patient's left eye. Simultaneously, apply a slight rapid increase of rotation of the head and neck to the left with no increase of sidebending to the right (Fig. 8.41). A key element in this technique is to avoid exaggeration of the primary leverage of sidebending when the thrust is applied. The use of sidebending as a primary leverage is predicated upon the operator's desire to limit the amount of head and neck rotation

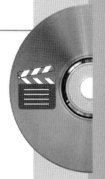

Cervical spine C2–7
Up-slope gliding

Patient sitting
Operator standing in front

Assume somatic dysfunction (S-T-A-R-T) is identified and you wish to use an upward and forward thrust, parallel to the apophysial joint plane, to produce joint cavitation at C4–5 on the left (Figs 8.42, 8.43).

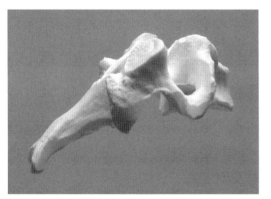

Figure 8.42

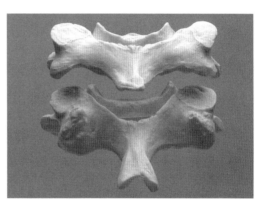

Figure 8.43

KEY

✳ Stabilization

● Applicator

➜ Plane of thrust (operator)

⇨ Direction of body movement (patient)

Note: The dimensions for the arrows are not a pictorial representation of the amplitude or force of the thrust.

1. **Contact point**

Posterolateral aspect of the left articular pillar of C4.

2. **Applicator**

Palmar aspect, proximal or middle phalanx of operator's right index or middle finger.

3. **Patient positioning**

Sitting with the neck in a neutral relaxed position. The neck should not be in any significant amount of flexion or extension.

4. **Operator stance**

Stand in front and to the right of the patient, feet spread slightly. Adjust couch height so that you can stand as erect as possible and

121

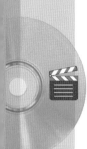

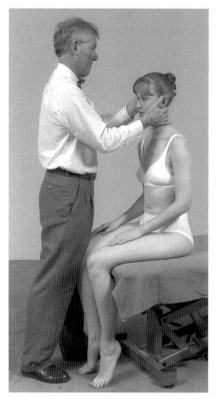

Figure 8.44

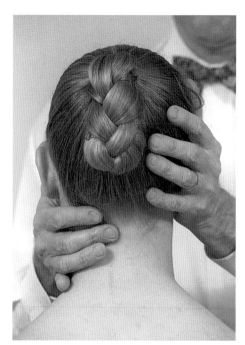

Figure 8.45

avoid crouching over the patient as this will limit the technique and restrict delivery of the thrust (Fig. 8.44).

5. Palpation of contact point

Place the fingers and palm of your left hand against the patient's right occiput and neck, gently covering the patient's right ear. Use the index or middle finger of your right hand to palpate the patient's left articular pillar of C4. Slowly but firmly slide your applicator along the articular pillar of C4 until it approximates the proximal or middle phalanx (Fig. 8.45). Several sliding pressures may be necessary to establish close approximation to the contact point.

6. Fixation of contact point

Keep your right index or middle finger firmly pressed upon the contact point while you spread the other fingers and thumb of the right hand to securely support the head, mandible and neck, thereby locking the applicator in

position. You must now keep the applicator on the contact point until the technique is complete. The weight of the head and neck is now balanced between your left and right hands, with the cervical spine positioning controlled by the converging pressures of your two hands.

7. Positioning for thrust

The elbows are held close to or only slightly away from your sides.

(a) *Primary leverage*. Ensure that the patient's head is securely supported between your two hands. Maintaining all holds and contact points, rotate the head and neck to the right until tension is palpated at the contact point (Fig. 8.46). Do not lose contact between your applicator and the articular pillar of C4. Do not force rotation; take it up fully but carefully. A common mistake is to use insufficient primary leverage of head and neck rotation.

(b) *Secondary leverage*. Add a very small degree of sidebending to the left, down to and including the C3–4 segment but leaving C4–5 free to move. *Note*: strong

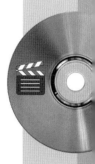

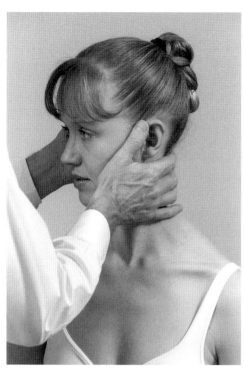

Figure 8.46

sidebending will lock the neck. Slight movements of the operator's forearms, shoulders and trunk introduce the sidebending.

8. Adjustments to achieve appropriate pre-thrust tension

Ensure your patient remains relaxed. It is important to keep your elbows close to your sides. Maintaining all holds, make any necessary changes in flexion, extension, sidebending or rotation until you can sense a state of appropriate tension and leverage. The patient should not be aware of any pain or discomfort. You make these final adjustments by slight movements of your legs and trunk, not by altering the position of the hands or arms.

9. Immediately pre-thrust

Relax and adjust your balance as necessary. Keep your head up; looking down impedes the thrust and can cause embarrassing proximity to the patient. An effective HVLA thrust technique is best achieved if both the operator and patient are relaxed and not holding

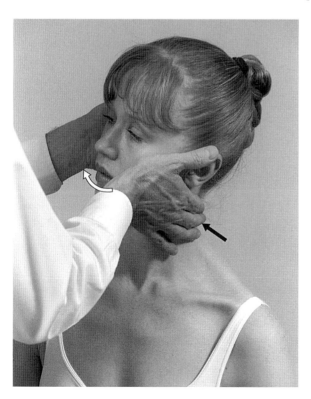

Figure 8.47

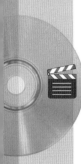

themselves rigid. This is a common impediment to achieving effective cavitation.

10. Delivering the thrust

Apply a HVLA thrust to the left articular pillar of C4. The thrust is upwards and towards the midline in the direction of the patient's right eye, parallel to the apophysial joint plane (Fig. 8.47). Simultaneously, apply a slight, rapid increase of rotation to the right, but do not increase sidebending leverages. This is a HVLA 'flick' type thrust. Coordination between the left and right hands and arms is critical.

The thrust, although very rapid, must never be excessively forcible. The aim should be to use the absolute minimum force necessary to achieve joint cavitation. A common fault arises from the use of excessive amplitude with insufficient velocity of thrust.

SUMMARY

Cervical spine C2–7 Up-slope gliding

Patient sitting

Operator standing in front

- **Contact point:** Posterolateral aspect of the left C4 articular pillar

- **Applicator:** Palmar aspect, proximal or middle phalanx

- **Patient positioning:** Sitting with the neck in a neutral relaxed position

- **Operator stance:** In front and to the right of the patient, feet spread slightly (Fig. 8.44)

- **Palpation of contact point**

- **Fixation of contact point:** Keep your right index or middle finger firmly pressed upon the contact point while you spread the other fingers and thumb of the right hand to securely support the head, mandible and neck (Fig. 8.45)

- **Positioning for thrust:** Stand upright with the elbows held close to or only slightly away from your sides. Introduce primary leverage of rotation to the right (Fig. 8.46) and a small degree of secondary leverage of sidebending left. Maintain the contact point on the posterolateral aspect of the C4 articular pillar

- **Adjustments to achieve appropriate pre-thrust tension**

- **Immediately pre-thrust:** Relax and adjust your balance

- **Delivering the thrust:** The thrust is directed towards the patient's right eye. Simultaneously, apply a slight, rapid increase of rotation of the head and neck to the right with no increase of sidebending to the left (Fig. 8.47). Coordination between both hands and arms is critical

8.10

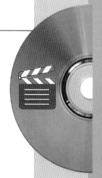

Cervical spine C2–7
Up-slope gliding

Patient sitting
Operator standing to the side

*Assume somatic dysfunction (S-T-A-R-T) is identified and you wish to use
an upward and forward gliding thrust, parallel to the apophysial joint plane,
to produce cavitation at C4–5 on the left (Figs. 8.48, 8.49).*

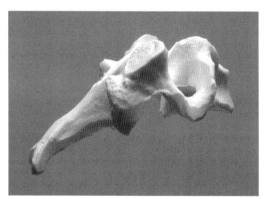

Figure 8.48

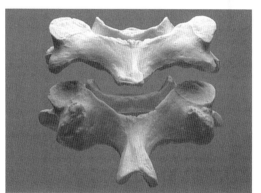

Figure 8.49

KEY

❋ Stabilization

● Applicator

→ Plane of thrust (operator)

⇨ Direction of body movement
(patient)

Note: The dimensions for the arrows are
not a pictorial representation of the
amplitude or force of the thrust.

1. **Contact point**

Posterolateral aspect of the left articular pillar
of C4.

2. **Applicator**

Palmar aspect, proximal or middle phalanx of
operator's right index or middle finger.

3. **Patient positioning**

Sitting with the neck in a neutral relaxed
position. The neck should not be in any
significant amount of flexion or extension.

4. **Operator stance**

Stand to the right of the patient, feet spread
slightly. Adjust couch height so that you can

125

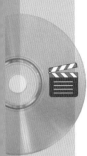

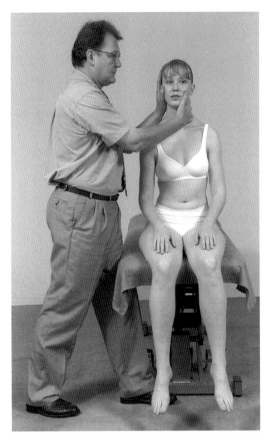

Figure 8.50

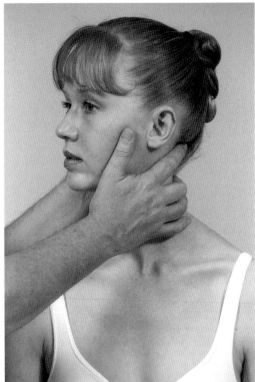

Figure 8.51

stand as erect as possible and avoid crouching over the patient as this will limit the technique and restrict delivery of the thrust (Fig. 8.50).

5. Palpation of contact point

Place the fingers and palm of your left hand over the right side of the patient's head and neck, gently covering the right ear. Reach in front of the patient with your right hand and palpate the left articular pillar of C4 with the tip of your right index or middle finger. Slowly but firmly slide your applicator along the articular pillar of C4 until it approximates the proximal or middle phalanx. Several sliding pressures may be necessary to establish close approximation to the contact point.

6. Fixation of contact point

Keep your right index or middle finger firmly pressed upon the contact point while you spread the other fingers and thumb of the right hand to securely support the head, mandible and neck, thereby locking the applicator in position. You must now keep the applicator on the contact point until the technique is complete. The weight of the head and neck is now balanced between your left and right hands, with the cervical spine positioning controlled by the converging pressures of your two hands.

7. Positioning for thrust

The elbows are held close to or only slightly away from your sides.

(a) *Primary leverage.* Ensure that the patient's head is securely supported between your two hands. Maintaining all holds and contact points, rotate the head and neck to the right until tension is palpated at the contact point (Fig. 8.51). Do not lose contact between your applicator and the articular pillar of C4. Do not force rotation; take it up fully but carefully. A common mistake is to use insufficient primary leverage of head and neck rotation.

(b) Secondary leverage. Add a very small degree of sidebending to the left, down to and including the C3–4 segment but leaving C4–5 free to move. Note: strong sidebending will lock the neck. Slight movements of the operator's forearms, shoulders and trunk introduce the sidebending.

8. Adjustments to achieve appropriate pre-thrust tension

Ensure your patient remains relaxed. It is important to keep your elbows close to your sides. Maintaining all holds, make any necessary changes in flexion, extension, sidebending or rotation until you can sense a state of appropriate tension and leverage. The patient should not be aware of any pain or discomfort. You make these final adjustments by slight movements of your legs and trunk, not by altering the position of the hands or arms.

9. Immediately pre-thrust

Relax and adjust your balance as necessary. Keep your head up; looking down impedes the thrust and can cause embarrassing proximity to the patient. An effective HVLA thrust technique is best achieved if both the operator and patient are relaxed and not holding themselves rigid. This is a common impediment to achieving effective cavitation.

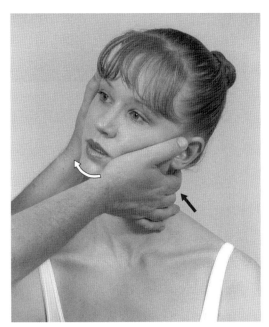

Figure 8.52

10. Delivering the thrust

Apply a HVLA thrust to the left articular pillar of C4. The thrust is upwards and towards the midline in the direction of the patient's right eye, parallel to the apophysial joint plane (Fig. 8.52). Simultaneously, apply a slight, rapid increase of rotation to the right, but do not increase sidebending leverages. This is a HVLA 'flick' type thrust. Coordination between the left and right hands and arms is critical.

The thrust, although very rapid, must never be excessively forcible. The aim should be to use the absolute minimum force necessary to achieve joint cavitation. A common fault arises from the use of excessive amplitude with insufficient velocity of thrust.

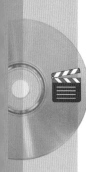

SUMMARY

Cervical spine C2–7 Up-slope gliding

Patient sitting

Operator standing to the side

- **Contact point:** Posterolateral aspect of the left C4 articular pillar
- **Applicator:** Palmar aspect, proximal or middle phalanx
- **Patient positioning:** Sitting with the neck in a neutral relaxed position
- **Operator stance:** To the right of the patient, feet spread slightly (Fig. 8.50)
- **Palpation of contact point**
- **Fixation of contact point**
- **Positioning for thrust:** Stand upright with the elbows held close to or only slightly away from your sides. Introduce primary leverage of rotation to the right (Fig. 8.51) and a small degree of secondary leverage of sidebending left. Maintain the contact point on the posterolateral aspect of the left C4 articular pillar
- **Adjustments to achieve appropriate pre-thrust tension**
- **Immediately pre-thrust:** Relax and adjust your balance
- **Delivering the thrust:** The thrust is directed towards the patient's right eye. Simultaneously, apply a slight, rapid increase of rotation of the head and neck to the right with no increase of sidebending left (Fig. 8.52). Coordination between both hands and arms is critical

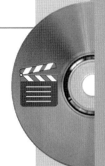

Cervical spine C2–7
Down-slope gliding

Chin hold
Patient supine

Assume somatic dysfunction (S-T-A-R-T) is identified and you wish to use a downward and backward gliding thrust, parallel to the apophysial joint plane, to produce cavitation at C4–5 on the right (Figs. 8.53, 8.54).

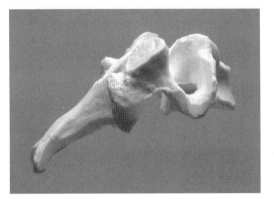

Figure 8.53

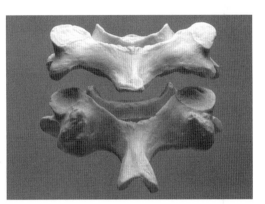

Figure 8.54

KEY

✳ Stabilization

● Applicator

➔ Plane of thrust (operator)

⇨ Direction of body movement (patient)

Note: The dimensions for the arrows are not a pictorial representation of the amplitude or force of the thrust.

1. Contact point

Lateral aspect of the right articular pillar of C4.

2. Applicator

Lateral border, proximal or middle phalanx of operator's right index finger.

3. Patient positioning

Supine with the neck in a neutral relaxed position. If necessary, remove pillow or adjust pillow height. The neck should not be in any significant amount of flexion or extension.

4. Operator stance

Head of couch, feet spread slightly. Adjust couch height so that you can stand as erect as possible and avoid crouching over the patient

129

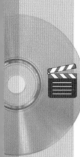

as this will limit the technique and restrict delivery of the thrust.

5. **Palpation of contact point**

Place fingers of both hands gently under the occiput. Rotate the head to the left, taking its weight in your left hand. Remove your right hand from the occiput and palpate the right articular pillar of C4 with the tip of your index or middle finger. Slowly but firmly slide your right index finger downwards (towards the couch) along the articular pillar until it approximates the middle or proximal phalanx. Several sliding pressures may be necessary to establish close approximation to the contact point.

6. **Fixation of contact point**

Keep your right index finger firmly pressed upon the contact point while you flex the other fingers and thumb of the right hand so as to clasp the back of the neck and thereby lock the applicator in position. You must now keep the applicator on the contact point until the technique is complete. Keeping the hands in position, return the head to the neutral position.

7. **Chin hold**

Keeping your right hand in position, slide the left hand slowly and carefully forwards until the fingers lightly clasp the chin. Ensure that your left forearm is over or slightly anterior to the ear. Placing the forearm on or behind the ear puts the neck into too much flexion. The head is now controlled by balancing forces between the right palm and left forearm. Maintain the applicator in position.

8. **Vertex contact**

Move your body forward slightly so that your chest is in contact with the vertex of the patient's head. The head is now securely cradled between your left forearm, the flexed left elbow, the right palm and your chest. Vertex contact is often useful in a heavy, stiff or difficult case but can, on occasions, be omitted.

9. **Positioning for thrust**

Step slightly to the right, keeping the hands firmly in position and taking care not to lose pressure on the contact point. This introduces an element of cervical sidebending to the right. Straighten your right wrist so that the radius and first metacarpal are in line. Align your body and right arm for the thrust plane, which is caudad in the direction of the patient's left shoulder and downwards towards the couch.

(a) Primary leverage of sidebending.
    Maintaining all holds and contact

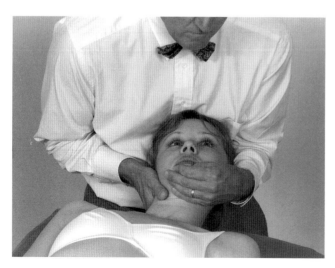

Figure 8.55

130

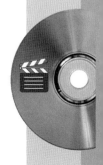

points, sidebend the patient's head and neck to the right until tension is palpated at the contact point (Fig. 8.55). The operator pivoting slightly, via the legs and trunk, introduces the right sidebending, so that the trunk and upper body rotate to the left, enabling the hands and arms to remain in position. Do not attempt to introduce sidebending by moving the hands or arms alone, as this will lead to loss of contact and inaccurate technique. Do not lose firm contact with your contact point on the articular pillar of C4. A common mistake is to use insufficient primary leverage of head and neck sidebending.

(b) *Secondary leverage.* Add a little rotation to the left, down to and including the C3–4 segment but leaving C4–5 free to move (Fig. 8.56). This requires extensive practice before one develops a refined 'tension sense'. Movement of your hands and forearms introduces the rotation.

10. **Adjustments to achieve appropriate pre-thrust tension**

Ensure your patient remains relaxed. Maintaining all holds, make any necessary changes in flexion, extension, sidebending or rotation until you can sense a state of appropriate tension and leverage. The patient should not be aware of any pain or discomfort. You make these final adjustments by slight movements of your ankles, knees, hips and trunk, not by altering the position of the hands or arms.

11. **Immediately pre-thrust**

Relax and adjust your balance as necessary. Keep your head up; looking down impedes the thrust and can cause embarrassing proximity to the patient. An effective HVLA thrust technique is best achieved if both the operator and patient are relaxed and not holding themselves rigid. This is a common impediment to achieving effective cavitation.

12. **Delivering the thrust**

Apply a HVLA thrust to the right articular pillar of C4. The direction of thrust is caudad in the direction of the patient's left shoulder and downwards towards the couch, parallel to the apophysial joint plane. Simultaneously, apply a slight, rapid increase of sidebending of the head and neck to the right but do not increase the rotation leverage (Fig. 8.57). The increase of sidebending is induced by a slight rotation of the operator's trunk and upper body to the left. A very rapid contraction of the flexors and adductors of the right shoulder joint induce

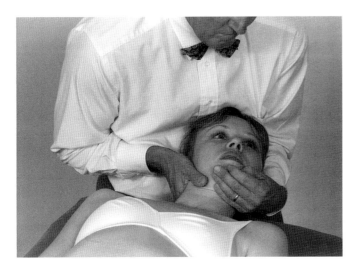

Figure 8.56

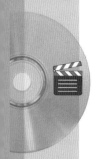

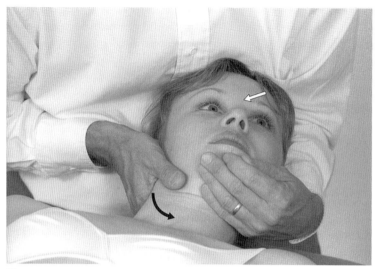

Figure 8.57

the thrust; if necessary, trunk and lower limb movement may be incorporated.

The thrust, although very rapid, must never be excessively forcible. The aim should be to use the absolute minimum force necessary to achieve joint cavitation. A common fault arises from the use of excessive amplitude with insufficient velocity of thrust.

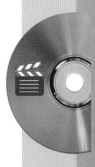

SUMMARY

Cervical spine C2–7 Down-slope gliding

Chin hold

Patient supine

- **Contact point:** Lateral aspect of the right C4 articular pillar
- **Applicator:** Lateral border, proximal or middle phalanx
- **Patient positioning:** Supine with the neck in a neutral relaxed position
- **Operator stance:** Head of couch, feet spread slightly
- **Palpation of contact point**
- **Fixation of contact point**
- **Chin hold:** Ensure your left forearm is over or slightly anterior to the ear
- **Vertex contact:** Optional but often useful
- **Positioning for thrust:** Step slightly to the right. Introduce primary leverage of sidebending right (Fig. 8.55) and a small degree of secondary leverage of rotation left (Fig. 8.56). Align your body and right arm for the thrust plane, which is caudad in the direction of the patient's left shoulder and downwards towards the couch
- **Adjustments to achieve appropriate pre-thrust tension**
- **Immediately pre-thrust:** Relax and adjust your balance
- **Delivering the thrust:** The thrust is directed towards the patient's left shoulder and downwards towards the couch. Simultaneously, apply a slight, rapid increase of sidebending of the head and neck to the right with no increase of rotation to the left (Fig. 8.57)

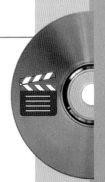

Cervical spine C2–7
Down-slope gliding

Cradle hold
Patient supine

Assume somatic dysfunction (S-T-A-R-T) is identified and you wish to use a downward and backward gliding thrust, parallel to the apophysial joint plane, to produce cavitation at C4–5 on the right (Figs 8.58, 8.59).

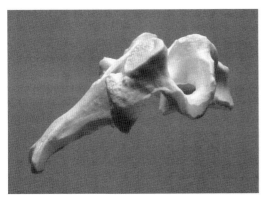

Figure 8.58

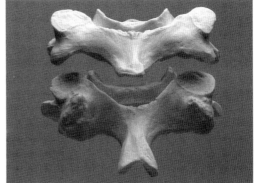

Figure 8.59

KEY

❋ Stabilization

● Applicator

→ Plane of thrust (operator)

⇨ Direction of body movement (patient)

Note: The dimensions for the arrows are not a pictorial representation of the amplitude or force of the thrust.

1. **Contact point**

The lateral aspect of the right articular pillar of C4.

2. **Applicator**

Lateral border, proximal or middle phalanx of operator's right index finger.

3. **Patient positioning**

Supine with the neck in a neutral relaxed position. If necessary, remove pillow or adjust pillow height. The neck should not be in any significant amount of flexion or extension.

4. **Operator stance**

Head of couch, feet spread slightly. Adjust couch height so that you can stand as erect as

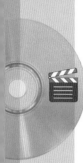

possible and avoid crouching over the patient as this will limit the technique and restrict delivery of the thrust.

5. Palpation of contact point

Place fingers of both hands gently under the occiput. Rotate the head to the left, taking its weight in your left hand. Remove your right hand from the occiput and palpate the right articular pillar of C4 with the tip of your index or middle finger. Slowly but firmly slide your right index finger downwards (towards the couch) along the articular pillar until it approximates the middle or proximal phalanx. Several sliding pressures may be necessary to establish close approximation to the contact point.

6. Fixation of contact point

Keep the right index finger firmly pressed on the contact point while you flex the other fingers and thumb of the right hand so as to clasp the back of the neck and thereby lock the applicator in position. You must now keep the applicator on the contact point until the technique is complete. Keeping the hands in position, return the head to the neutral position.

7. Cradle hold

Keep the left hand under the head and spread the fingers out for maximum contact; keep the patient's ear resting in the palm of the your left hand. Flex the left wrist, allowing you to cradle the patient's head in your palm, flexed wrist and anterior aspect of forearm. Keep your right index finger firmly on the contact point and press the right palm against the occiput. The weight of the patient's head and neck is now balanced between your left and right hands, with the cervical positioning controlled by the converging pressures of your two hands and arms. When treating the lower cervical segments, the middle or distal phalanx may be used as the applicator.

8. Vertex contact

None in this technique.

9. Positioning for thrust

The elbows are held close to or only slightly away from your sides. This is an essential feature of the cradle hold method. Stand easily upright at the head of the couch and do not step to the right as in the chin hold method.

(a) *Primary leverage of sidebending.* Maintaining all holds and contact points, gently introduce sidebending of the head and neck to the right until tension is palpated at the contact point (Fig. 8.60). To introduce the right sidebending, the operator pivots slightly via the legs and trunk so that the trunk and upper body rotate to the left, enabling the hands and arms to remain in position. Do not lose firm contact with your contact point on the articular pillar of C4. A common mistake is to use insufficient primary leverage of head and neck sidebending.

(b) *Secondary leverage.* Add a little rotation to the left, down to and including the C3–4 segment but leaving C4–5 free to move

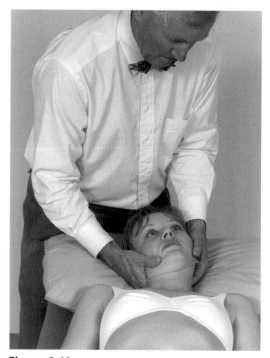

Figure 8.60

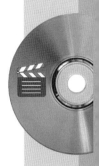

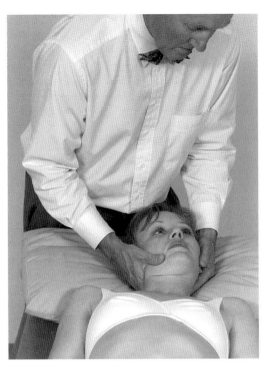

Figure 8.61

(Fig. 8.61). This requires extensive practice before one develops a refined 'tension sense'. Movement of your hands and forearms introduces the rotation.

10. Adjustments to achieve appropriate pre-thrust tension

Ensure your patient remains relaxed. Maintaining all holds, make any necessary changes in flexion, extension, sidebending or rotation until you can sense a state of appropriate tension and leverage. The patient should not be aware of any pain or discomfort. You make these final adjustments by slight movements of your ankles, knees, hips and trunk, not by altering the position of the hands or arms.

11. Immediately pre-thrust

Relax and adjust your balance as necessary. Keep your head up; looking down impedes the thrust and can cause embarrassing proximity to the patient. An effective HVLA thrust technique is best achieved if both the operator and patient are relaxed and not holding themselves rigid. This is a common impediment to achieving effective cavitation.

Ensure the patient's head and neck remain on the pillow as this facilitates the arrest of the technique and limits excessive amplitude of thrust.

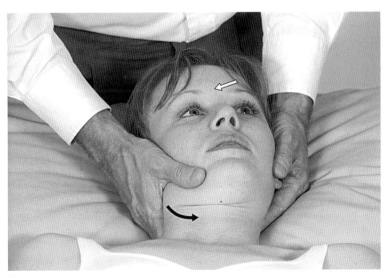

Figure 8.62

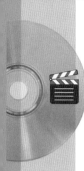

Note that the final thrust is directed in a downward and backward direction parallel to the facet joint plane. The thrust is directed towards the patient's left shoulder as illustrated. The primary leverage is sidebending to the right and the secondary (lesser leverage) is rotation to the left.

12. Delivering the thrust

Apply a HVLA thrust to the right articular pillar of C4. The direction of thrust is caudad in the direction of the patient's left shoulder and downwards towards the couch, parallel to the apophysial joint plane (Fig. 8.62). The operator rotating the trunk and upper body to the left, enabling the hands and arms to remain in position on the cervical spine, generates the thrust. Simultaneously, apply a very slight, rapid increase of sidebending of the head and neck to the right but do not increase the rotation leverage.

The thrust, although very rapid, must never be excessively forcible. The aim should be to use the absolute minimum force necessary to achieve joint cavitation. A common fault arises from the use of excessive amplitude with insufficient velocity of thrust.

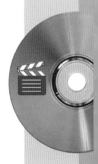

SUMMARY

Cervical spine C2–7 Down-slope gliding

Cradle hold

Patient supine

- **Contact point:** Lateral aspect of the right C4 articular pillar
- **Applicator:** Lateral border, proximal or middle phalanx
- **Patient positioning:** Supine with the neck in a neutral relaxed position
- **Operator stance:** Head of couch, feet spread slightly
- **Palpation of contact point**
- **Fixation of contact point**
- **Cradle hold:** The weight of the patient's head and neck is balanced between your left and right hands with cervical positioning controlled by the converging pressures
- **Vertex contact:** None
- **Positioning for thrust:** Stand upright at the head of the couch. The elbows are held close to or only slightly away from your sides. Introduce primary leverage of sidebending to the right (Fig. 8.60) and a small degree of secondary leverage of rotation left (Fig. 8.61). Maintain the contact point on the lateral aspect of the right C4 articular pillar
- **Adjustments to achieve appropriate pre-thrust tension**
- **Immediately pre-thrust:** Relax and adjust your balance
- **Delivering the thrust:** The thrust is directed towards the patient's left shoulder and downwards towards the couch. Simultaneously, apply a slight, rapid increase of sidebending of the head and neck to the right with no increase of rotation to the left (Fig. 8.62)

139

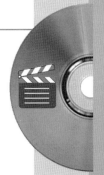

Cervical spine C2–7
Down-slope gliding

Patient sitting
Operator standing to the side

Assume somatic dysfunction (S-T-A-R-T) is identified and you wish to use a downward and backward gliding thrust, parallel to the apophysial joint plane, to produce cavitation at C4–5 on the right (Figs 8.63, 8.64).

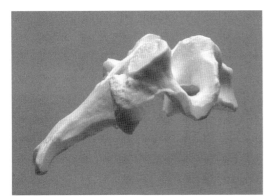

Figure 8.63

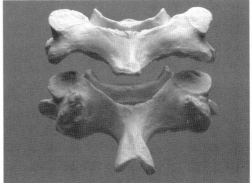

Figure 8.64

KEY

❊ Stabilization

● Applicator

→ Plane of thrust (operator)

⇨ Direction of body movement (patient)

Note: The dimensions for the arrows are not a pictorial representation of the amplitude or force of the thrust.

1. **Contact point**

Lateral aspect of the right articular pillar of C4.

2. **Applicator**

Palmar aspect, proximal or middle phalanx of operator's left index or middle finger.

3. **Patient positioning**

Sitting with the neck in a neutral relaxed position. The neck should not be in any significant amount of flexion or extension.

4. **Operator stance**

Stand to the left of the patient, feet spread slightly. Adjust couch height so that you can stand as erect as possible and avoid crouching

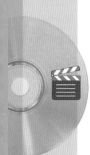

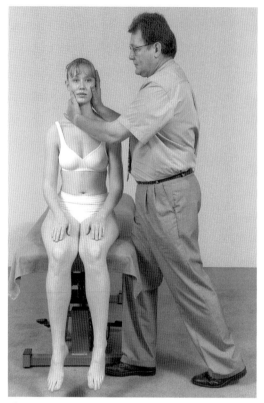

Figure 8.65

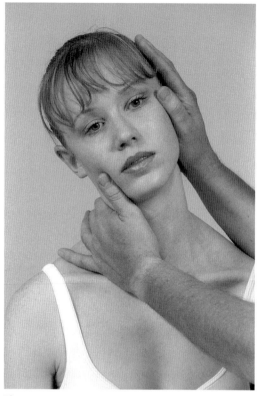

Figure 8.66

over the patient as this will limit the technique and restrict delivery of the thrust (Fig. 8.65).

5. Palpation of contact point

Place the fingers and palm of your right hand over the left side of the patient's head and neck, gently covering the left ear. Reach in front of the patient with your left hand and palpate the right articular pillar of C4 with the tip of your left index or middle finger. Slowly but firmly slide your applicator along the articular pillar of C4 until it approximates the proximal or middle phalanx. Several sliding pressures may be necessary to establish close approximation to the contact point.

6. Fixation of contact point

Keep your left index or middle finger firmly pressed upon the contact point while you spread the other fingers and thumb of the left

hand to securely support the head, mandible and neck, thereby locking the applicator in position. You must now keep the applicator on the contact point until the technique is complete. The weight of the head and neck is now balanced between your right and left hands, with the cervical spine positioning controlled by the converging pressures of your two hands.

7. Positioning for thrust

The elbows are held close to or only slightly away from your sides.

(a) *Primary leverage.* Ensure that the patient's head is securely supported between your two hands. Maintaining all holds and contact points, sidebend the head and neck to the right until tension is palpated at the contact point (Fig. 8.66). Do not lose contact between your applicator and

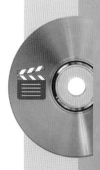

the articular pillar of C4. Do not force sidebending; take it up fully but carefully. A common mistake is to use insufficient primary leverage of head and neck sidebending.

(b) *Secondary leverage.* Add a very small degree of rotation to the left, down to and including the C3–4 segment but leaving C4–5 free to move. Slight movements of the operator's hands and arms introduce the rotation.

8. Adjustments to achieve appropriate pre-thrust tension

Ensure your patient remains relaxed. It is important to keep your elbows close to your sides. Maintaining all holds, make any necessary changes in flexion, extension, sidebending or rotation until you can sense a state of appropriate tension and leverage. The patient should not be aware of any pain or discomfort.

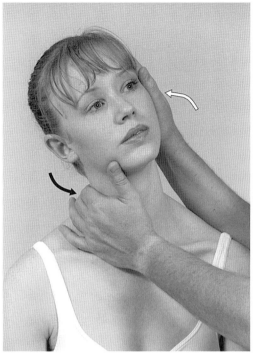

Figure 8.67

9. Immediately pre-thrust

Relax and adjust your balance as necessary. Keep your head up; looking down impedes the thrust and can cause embarrassing proximity to the patient. An effective HVLA thrust technique is best achieved if both the operator and patient are relaxed and not holding themselves rigid. This is a common impediment to achieving effective cavitation.

10. Delivering the thrust

Apply a HVLA thrust to the right articular pillar of C4. The thrust is caudad and towards the

patient's left shoulder, parallel to the apophysial joint plane (Fig. 8.67). Simultaneously, apply a slight, rapid increase of sidebending to the right but do not increase rotation leverage. This is a HVLA 'flick' type thrust. Coordination between the left and right hands and arms is critical.

The thrust, although very rapid, must never be excessively forcible. The aim should be to use the absolute minimum force necessary to achieve joint cavitation. A common fault arises from the use of excessive amplitude with insufficient velocity of thrust.

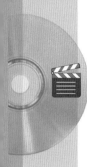

SUMMARY

Cervical spine C2–7 Down-slope gliding

Patient sitting

Operator standing to the side

- **Contact point:** Lateral aspect of the right C4 articular pillar
- **Applicator:** Palmar aspect, proximal or middle phalanx
- **Patient positioning:** Sitting with the neck in a neutral relaxed position
- **Operator stance:** To the left of the patient, feet spread slightly (Fig. 8.65)
- **Palpation of contact point**
- **Fixation of contact point**
- **Positioning for thrust:** Stand upright with the elbows held close to or only slightly away from your sides. Introduce primary leverage of sidebending to the right (Fig. 8.66) and a small degree of secondary leverage of rotation left. Maintain the contact point on the lateral aspect of the right C4 articular pillar
- **Adjustments to achieve appropriate pre-thrust tension**
- **Immediately pre-thrust:** Relax and adjust your balance
- **Delivering the thrust:** The thrust is caudad and towards the patient's left shoulder. Simultaneously, apply a slight, rapid increase of sidebending of the head and neck to the right with no increase of rotation to the left (Fig. 8.67). Coordination between both hands and arms is critical

8.14

Cervicothoracic spine C7–T3
Rotation gliding

Patient prone
Operator at side of couch

Assume somatic dysfunction (S-T-A-R-T) is identified and you wish to use a rotation gliding thrust, parallel to the apophysial joint plane, to produce cavitation at the T2–3 apophysial joint (Figs 8.68, 8.69).

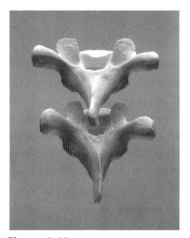

Figure 8.68

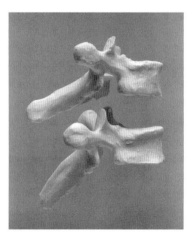

Figure 8.69

1. Contact point

Right side of spinous process of T3.

2. Applicator

Thumb of right hand.

3. Patient positioning

Patient lying prone with the head and neck turned to the left and arms hanging over the edge of the couch or against the patient's sides (Fig. 8.70). Introduce a small amount of sidebending to the right by gently moving the patient's head to the right while in the rotated position. Do not introduce too much sidebending.

KEY

✳ Stabilization

● Applicator

→ Plane of thrust (operator)

⇨ Direction of body movement (patient)

Note: The dimensions for the arrows are not a pictorial representation of the amplitude or force of the thrust.

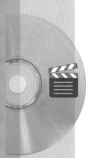

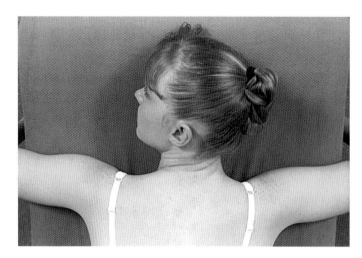

Figure 8.70

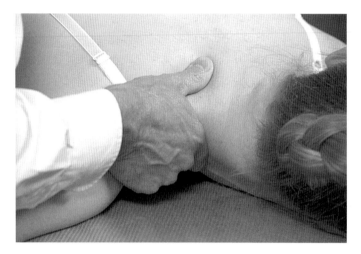

Figure 8.71

4. Operator stance

Stand on the right side of the patient facing towards the head of the couch.

5. Palpation of contact point

Locate the spinous process of T3. Place the thumb of your right hand gently but firmly against the right side of this spinous process. Spread the fingers of your right hand to rest over the patient's right trapezius muscle with your fingertips resting on the patient's right clavicle (Fig. 8.71). Ensure that you have good contact and will not slip off the spinous process of T3 when you apply a force against it. Maintain this contact point.

6. Positioning for thrust

Keeping your position at the side of the couch, gently place your left hand against the left side of the patient's head. This hand will control the rotation and sidebending leverages. Increase rotation of the patient's head and neck to the left by applying gentle pressure to the patient's head until a sense of tension is palpated at the contact point. Move your right forearm so that it lines up with your thumb against the spinous process of T3 and forms an angle of approximately 90° at the elbow (Fig. 8.72).

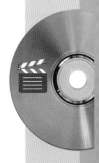

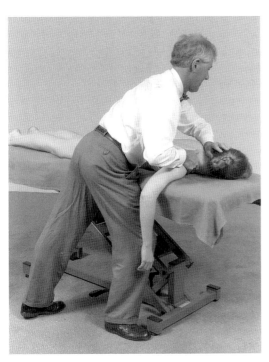

Figure 8.72

7. Adjustments to achieve appropriate pre-thrust tension

Ensure the patient remains relaxed. Maintaining all holds, make any necessary changes in extension, sidebending or rotation until you can sense a state of appropriate tension and leverage. The patient should not be aware of any pain or discomfort. Make these final adjustments by altering the pressure and direction of forces between the left hand against the patient's head and your right thumb at the contact point.

8. Immediately pre-thrust

Relax and adjust your balance as necessary. Keep your head up and ensure that your contacts are firm and your body position is well controlled. An effective HVLA thrust technique is best achieved if the operator and patient are relaxed and not holding themselves rigid. This is a common impediment to achieving effective cavitation.

9. Delivering the thrust

Apply a HVLA thrust to the spinous process of T3 in the direction of the patient's left shoulder joint. Simultaneously, apply a slight, rapid increase of head and neck rotation to the left with your left hand (Fig. 8.73). The thrust induces local rotation of the T3 vertebra, focusing forces at the T2–3 segment. You must not overemphasize

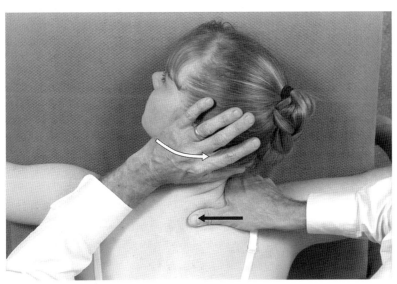

Figure 8.73

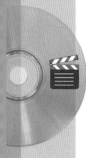

the thrust with your left hand against the patient's head. Your left hand stabilizes the leverages and maintains the position of the head against the thrust imposed upon the contact point. The thrust is induced by a very rapid contraction of the shoulder adductors.

The thrust, although very rapid, must never be excessively forcible. The aim should be to use the absolute minimum force necessary to achieve joint cavitation. A common fault arises from the use of excessive amplitude with insufficient velocity of thrust.

SUMMARY

Cervicothoracic spine C7–T3 Rotation gliding

Patient prone

Operator at side of couch

- **Contact point:** Right side of T3 spinous process

- **Applicator:** Thumb of right hand

- **Patient positioning:** Prone with the head rotated to the left and arms hanging over the edge of the couch or against the patient's sides (Fig. 8.70). Introduce a small amount of sidebending to the right. Do not introduce too much sidebending

- **Operator stance:** Right side of the patient facing towards the head of the couch

- **Palpation of contact point:** Place the thumb of your right hand against the right side of the spinous process of T3. Spread the fingers of your right hand to rest over the patient's trapezius muscle and clavicle (Fig. 8.71)

- **Positioning for thrust:** Place your left hand against the left side of the patient's head. Increase rotation of the head and neck to the left until a sense of tension is palpated at the contact point. Move your right forearm so that it lines up with your thumb against the spinous process of T3 and forms an angle of approximately 90° at the elbow (Fig. 8.72)

- **Adjustments to achieve appropriate pre-thrust tension**

- **Immediately pre-thrust:** Relax and adjust your balance

- **Delivering the thrust:** Thrust is directed towards the patient's left shoulder joint. Simultaneously, apply a slight rapid increase of head and neck rotation to the left with your left hand (Fig. 8.73). You must not overemphasize the thrust with your left hand against the patient's head

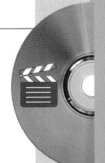

8.15

Cervicothoracic spine C7–T3
Rotation gliding

Patient prone
Operator at head of couch

Assume somatic dysfunction (S-T-A-R-T) is identified and you wish to use a rotation gliding thrust, parallel to the apophysial joint plane, to produce cavitation at the T2–3 apophysial joint (Figs 8.74, 8.75).

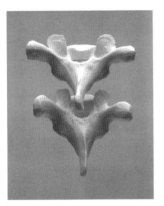

Figure 8.74

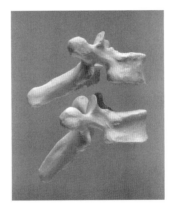

Figure 8.75

KEY

✳ Stabilization

● Applicator

→ Plane of thrust (operator)

⇨ Direction of body movement
(patient)

Note: The dimensions for the arrows are
not a pictorial representation of the
amplitude or force of the thrust.

1. **Contact point**

Transverse process of T3 on the left.

2. **Applicator**

Hypothenar eminence of left hand.

3. **Patient positioning**

Patient prone with the point of the chin resting
on the couch and the arms hanging over the
edge of the couch or against the patient's sides.
Introduce a small amount of sidebending to
the right by gently lifting and moving the
patient's chin to the right (Fig. 8.76). Do not
introduce too much sidebending.

4. **Operator stance**

Head of the couch, feet spread slightly. Stand
as erect as possible and avoid crouching over

149

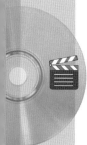

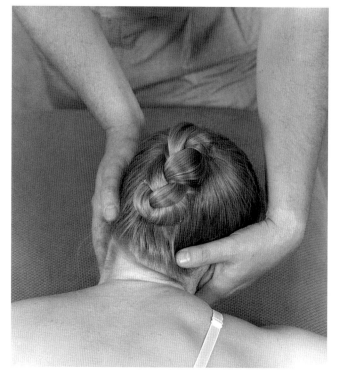

Figure 8.76

the patient as this will limit the technique and restrict delivery of the thrust.

5. **Palpation of contact point**

Locate the transverse process of T3 on the left. Place the hypothenar eminence of your left hand gently but firmly against the transverse process of T3 on the left. Ensure that you have good contact and will not slip across the skin or superficial musculature when you apply a caudad and downward force towards the couch against the transverse process of T3. Maintain this contact point.

6. **Positioning for thrust**

Keeping your position at the head of the couch, gently place your right hand against the left side of the patient's head and neck with your fingers pointing towards the patient's right shoulder. While maintaining the right sidebending introduced earlier, begin to rotate the cervical and upper thoracic spine to the left by applying gentle pushing pressure to the left side of the patient's head and neck with your right hand (Fig. 8.77). Maintaining all holds

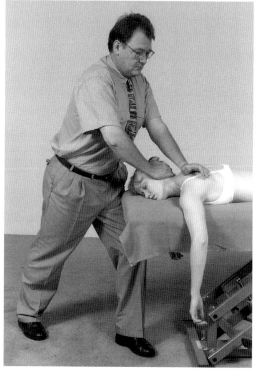

Figure 8.77

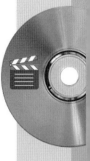

and pressures, complete the rotation of the patient's head and neck until a sense of tension is palpated at your left hypothenar eminence. Keep firm pressure against the contact point.

7. **Adjustments to achieve appropriate pre-thrust tension**

Ensure the patient remains relaxed. Maintaining all holds, make any necessary changes in extension, sidebending or rotation until you can sense a state of appropriate tension and leverage. The patient should not be aware of any pain or discomfort. You make these final adjustments by altering the pressure and direction of forces between the right hand against the patient's head and neck and your left hypothenar eminence against the contact point.

8. **Immediately pre-thrust**

Relax and adjust your balance as necessary. Keep your head up and ensure that your contacts are firm and that your body position is well controlled. An effective HVLA thrust technique is best achieved if the operator and patient are relaxed and not

holding themselves rigid. This is a common impediment to achieving effective cavitation.

9. **Delivering the thrust**

Apply a HVLA thrust to the left transverse process of T3 down towards the couch and in the direction of the patient's left axilla. Simultaneously, apply a slight, rapid increase of head and neck rotation to the left with your right hand (Fig. 8.78). The thrust induces local rotation of the T3 vertebra, focusing forces at the T2–3 segment. You must not overemphasize the thrust with your right hand against the patient's head and neck. Your right hand stabilizes the leverages and maintains the position of the head and cervical spine against the thrust imposed upon the contact point. The thrust is induced by a very rapid contraction of the triceps, shoulder adductors and internal rotators.

The thrust, although very rapid, must never be excessively forcible. The aim should be to use the absolute minimum force necessary to achieve joint cavitation. A common fault arises from the use of excessive amplitude with insufficient velocity of thrust.

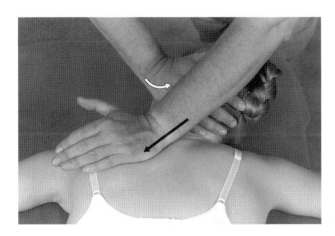

Figure 8.78

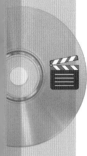

SUMMARY

Cervicothoracic spine C7–T3 Rotation gliding

Patient prone

Operator at head of couch

- **Contact point:** Left T3 transverse process

- **Applicator:** Hypothenar eminence of the left hand

- **Patient positioning:** Patient prone with the chin resting on the couch and the arms hanging over the edge of the couch or against the patient's sides. Introduce sidebending to the right (Fig. 8.76). Do not introduce too much sidebending

- **Operator stance:** Head of the couch, feet spread slightly

- **Palpation of contact point:** Place your hypothenar eminence against the transverse process of T3 on the left

- **Positioning for thrust:** Place your right hand against the left side of the patient's head and neck. Rotate the cervical and upper thoracic spine to the left by applying pushing pressure to the left side of the patient's head and neck with your right hand until a sense of tension is palpated at the contact point (Fig. 8.77)

- **Adjustments to achieve appropriate pre-thrust tension**

- **Immediately pre-thrust:** Relax and adjust your balance

- **Delivering the thrust:** The thrust is in the direction of the patient's left axilla and down towards the couch. Simultaneously, apply a slight rapid increase of head and neck rotation to the left with your right hand (Fig. 8.78). You must not overemphasize the thrust with your right hand against the patient's head

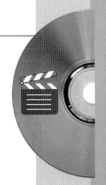

Cervicothoracic spine C7–T3
Rotation gliding

Patient prone
Operator at head of couch – variation

Assume somatic dysfunction (S-T-A-R-T) is identified and you wish to use a rotation gliding thrust, parallel to the apophysial joint plane, to produce cavitation at the T2–3 apophysial joint (Figs 8.79, 8.80).

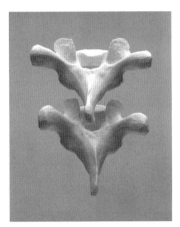

Figure 8.79

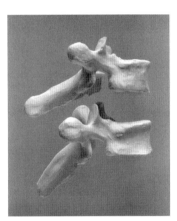

Figure 8.80

KEY

✳ Stabilization

● Applicator

→ Plane of thrust (operator)

⇨ Direction of body movement (patient)

Note: The dimensions for the arrows are not a pictorial representation of the amplitude or force of the thrust.

1. **Contact point**

Transverse process of T3 on the left.

2. **Applicator**

Hypothenar eminence of left hand.

3. **Patient positioning**

Patient prone with the point of the chin resting on the couch and the arms hanging over the edge of the couch or against the patient's sides. Introduce slight head and neck flexion. Now introduce a small amount of sidebending to the right by gently lifting and moving the patient's head to the right (Fig. 8.81).

4. **Operator stance**

To the right of the head of the couch, feet spread slightly. Stand as erect as possible and

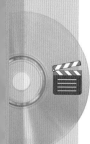

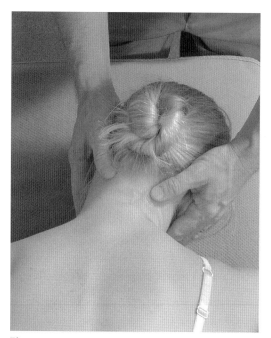

Figure 8.81

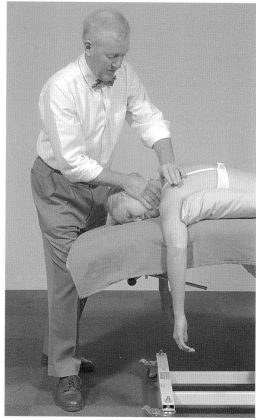

Figure 8.82

avoid crouching over the patient as this will limit the technique and restrict delivery of the thrust.

5. **Palpation of contact point**

Locate the transverse process of T3 on the left. Place the hypothenar eminence of your left hand gently but firmly against the transverse process of T3 on the left. Ensure that you have good contact and will not slip across the skin or superficial musculature when you apply a caudad and downward force towards the couch against the transverse process of T3. Maintain this contact point.

6. **Positioning for thrust**

Keeping your position at the head of the couch, gently place your right hand against the left side of the patient's head and neck with your fingers pointing towards the couch. While maintaining the right sidebending introduced earlier, begin to rotate the cervical and upper thoracic spine to the left by applying gentle pulling pressure to the left side of the patient's head and neck with your right hand (Fig. 8.82). Maintaining all holds and

pressures, complete the rotation of the patient's head and neck until a sense of tension is palpated at your left hypothenar eminence. Keep firm pressure against the contact point.

7. **Adjustments to achieve appropriate pre-thrust tension**

Ensure the patient remains relaxed. Maintaining all holds, make any necessary changes in flexion, extension, sidebending or rotation until you can sense a state of appropriate tension and leverage. The patient should not be aware of any pain or discomfort. You make these final adjustments by altering the pressure and direction of forces between the right hand against the patient's head and neck and your left hypothenar eminence against the contact point.

8. **Immediately pre-thrust**

Relax and adjust your balance as necessary. Keep your head up and ensure that your contacts are firm and that your body position is well controlled. An effective HVLA thrust technique is best achieved if the operator and patient are relaxed and not holding themselves rigid. This is a common impediment to achieving effective cavitation.

9. **Delivering the thrust**

Apply a HVLA thrust to the left transverse process of T3 down towards the couch and in the direction of the patient's left axilla. Simultaneously, apply a slight, rapid increase of head and neck rotation to the left with your right hand (Fig. 8.83). The thrust induces local rotation of the T3 vertebra, focusing forces at the T2–3 segment. You must not overemphasize the thrust with your right hand against the patient's head and neck. Your right hand stabilizes the leverages and maintains the position of the head and cervical spine against the thrust imposed upon the contact point. The thrust is induced by a very rapid contraction of the triceps, shoulder adductors and internal rotators.

The thrust, although very rapid, must never be excessively forcible. The aim should be to use the absolute minimum force necessary to achieve joint cavitation. A common fault arises from the use of excessive amplitude with insufficient velocity of thrust.

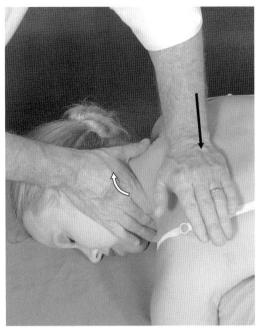
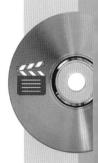

Figure 8.83

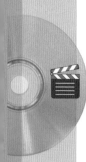

SUMMARY

Cervicothoracic spine C7–T3 Rotation gliding

Patient prone

Operator at head of couch

- **Contact point:** Left T3 transverse process

- **Applicator:** Hypothenar eminence of the left hand

- **Patient positioning:** Patient prone with the chin resting on the couch and the arms hanging over the edge of the couch or against the patient's sides. Introduce slight head and neck flexion. Introduce sidebending to the right (Fig. 8.81). Do not introduce too much sidebending

- **Operator stance:** To the right of the head of the couch, feet spread slightly

- **Palpation of contact point:** Place your hypothenar eminence against the transverse process of T3 on the left

- **Positioning for thrust:** Place your right hand against the left side of the patient's head and neck with your fingers pointing towards the couch. Rotate the cervical and upper thoracic spine to the left by applying pulling pressure to the left side of the patient's head and neck with your right hand until a sense of tension is palpated at the contact point (Fig. 8.82)

- **Adjustments to achieve appropriate pre-thrust tension**

- **Immediately pre-thrust:** Relax and adjust your balance

- **Delivering the thrust:** The thrust is in the direction of the patient's left axilla and down towards the couch. Simultaneously, apply a slight rapid increase of head and neck rotation to the left with your right hand (Fig. 8.83). You must not overemphasize the thrust with your right hand against the patient's head

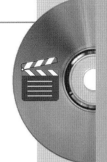

Cervicothoracic spine C7–T3
Sidebending gliding

Patient sitting

Assume somatic dysfunction (S-T-A-R-T) is identified and you wish to use a sidebending gliding thrust, parallel to the apophysial joint plane, to produce cavitation at the T2–3 apophysial joint (Figs 8.84, 8.85).

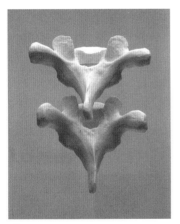

Figure 8.84

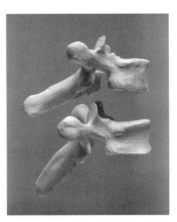

Figure 8.85

KEY

✳ Stabilization

● Applicator

→ Plane of thrust (operator)

⇨ Direction of body movement (patient)

Note: The dimensions for the arrows are not a pictorial representation of the amplitude or force of the thrust.

1. **Contact point**

Left side of the spinous process of T2.

2. **Applicator**

Thumb of left hand.

3. **Patient positioning**

Patient sitting with back towards the operator.

4. **Operator stance**

Stand behind the patient.

5. **Palpation of contact point**

Locate the spinous process of T2. Place the thumb of your left hand gently but firmly against the left side of this spinous process.

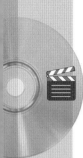

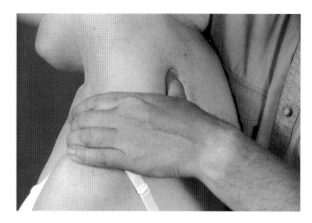

Figure 8.86

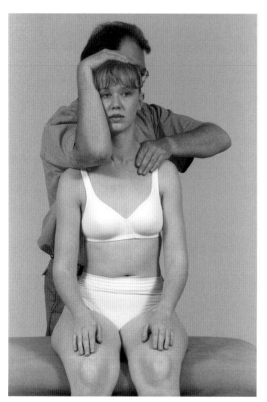

Figure 8.87

Spread the fingers of your left hand to rest over the patient's left trapezius muscle with your fingertips resting on the patient's left clavicle (Fig. 8.86). Ensure that you have good contact and will not slip off the spinous process of T2 when you apply a force against it. Maintain this contact point.

6. Positioning for thrust

Keeping your position behind the patient place your right hand and forearm alongside the right side of the patient's head and neck and gently rest the palm of your hand over the top of the patient's head (Fig. 8.87). Ensure that your forearm remains anterior to, and just over, the patient's ear. This hand will introduce and control the rotation and sidebending leverages.

Use your left hand to slightly rotate the patient's trunk to the left while using your right hand to introduce head and neck rotation to the right until a sense of tension is palpated at the contact point (Fig. 8.88). Now gently introduce cervical sidebending to the left by allowing the patient's body weight to fall slightly to the right. Keeping the patient's head centred over the sacrum, guide the neck into left sidebending with your right arm against the right side of the patient's head. A vertex compression force can be added to assist in localizing forces to the T2–3 segment. Ensure that your applicator thumb forms a straight line with your left forearm.

7. Adjustments to achieve appropriate pre-thrust tension

Ensure the patient remains relaxed. Maintaining all holds, make any necessary changes in flexion, extension, sidebending or rotation until you can sense a state of appropriate tension and leverage. The patient

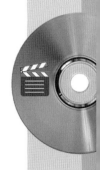

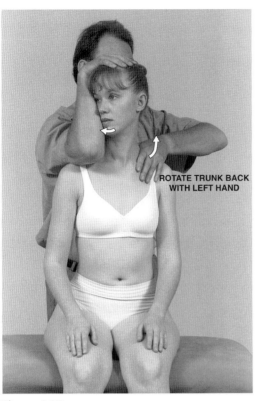

ROTATE TRUNK BACK
WITH LEFT HAND

Figure 8.88

should not be aware of any pain or discomfort. Make these final adjustments by balancing the pressure and direction of forces between the left hand against the contact point and the right hand and forearm against the patient's head and neck.

8. **Immediately pre-thrust**

Relax and adjust your balance as necessary. Keep your head up and ensure that your contacts are firm and that the patient's body weight and position are well controlled. An effective HVLA thrust technique is best achieved if the operator and patient are relaxed and not holding themselves rigid. This is a common impediment to achieving effective cavitation.

9. **Delivering the thrust**

Apply a HVLA thrust to the left side of the spinous process of T2 in the direction of the patient's right axilla. At the same time, slightly increase head and neck sidebending to the left with your right arm (Fig. 8.89). The thrust on the spinous

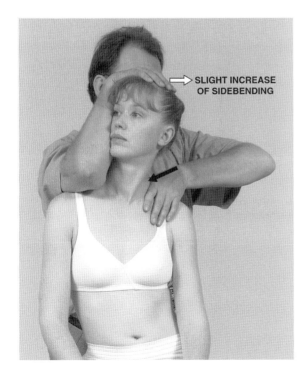

SLIGHT INCREASE
OF SIDEBENDING

Figure 8.89

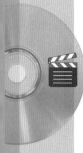

process of T2 and the slight increase in neck sidebending to the left focus forces at the T2–3 segment and causes cavitation at that level. The thrust is induced by a very rapid contraction of the shoulder adductors.

The thrust, although very rapid, must never be excessively forcible. The aim should be to use the absolute minimum force necessary to achieve joint cavitation. A common fault arises from the use of excessive amplitude with insufficient velocity of thrust.

SUMMARY

Cervicothoracic spine C7–T3 Sidebending gliding

Patient sitting

- **Contact point:** Left side of the T2 spinous process

- **Applicator:** Thumb of left hand

- **Patient positioning:** Patient sitting with back towards the operator

- **Operator stance:** Behind the patient

- **Palpation of contact point:** Place your left thumb against the left side of the T2 spinous process. Spread the fingers of your left hand to rest over the patient's trapezius muscle and clavicle (Fig. 8.86)

- **Positioning for thrust:** Place your right hand and forearm alongside the right side of the patient's head and neck (Fig. 8.87). Use your left hand to slightly rotate the patient's trunk to the left whilst using your right hand to introduce head and neck rotation to the right (Fig. 8.88). Introduce left sidebending to the cervical spine, localizing forces to the T2–3 segment. Ensure that your applicator thumb forms a straight line with your left forearm

- **Adjustments to achieve appropriate pre-thrust tension**

- **Immediately pre-thrust:** Relax and adjust your balance

- **Delivering the thrust:** The thrust is directed towards the patient's right axilla. Simultaneously, apply a slight, rapid increase of head and neck sidebending to the left (Fig. 8.89)

Cervicothoracic spine C7–T3
Sidebending gliding

Patient sitting
Ligamentous myofascial tension locking

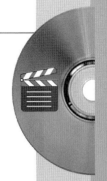

Assume somatic dysfunction (S-T-A-R-T) is identified and you wish to use a sidebending gliding thrust, parallel to the apophysial joint plane, to produce cavitation at the T2–3 apophysial joint (Figs 8.90, 8.91).

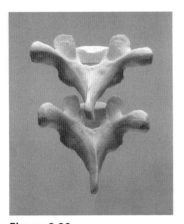

Figure 8.90

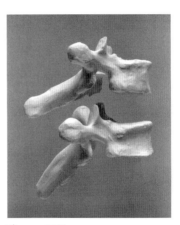

Figure 8.91

KEY

✳ Stabilization

● Applicator

→ Plane of thrust (operator)

⇨ Direction of body movement (patient)

Note: The dimensions for the arrows are not a pictorial representation of the amplitude or force of the thrust.

---

1. **Contact point**

Left side of the spinous process of T2.

2. **Applicator**

Thumb of left hand.

3. **Patient positioning**

Patient sitting with back towards the operator.

4. **Operator stance**

Stand behind the patient.

5. **Palpation of contact point**

Locate the spinous process of T2. Place the thumb of your left hand gently but firmly against the left side of this spinous process.

161

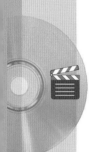

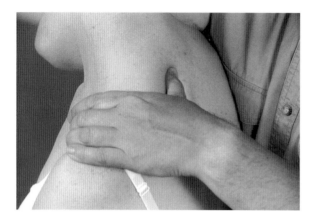

Figure 8.92

Spread the fingers of your left hand to rest over the patient's left trapezius muscle with your fingertips resting on the patient's left clavicle (Fig. 8.92). Ensure that you have good contact and will not slip off the spinous process of T2 when you apply a force against it. Maintain this contact point.

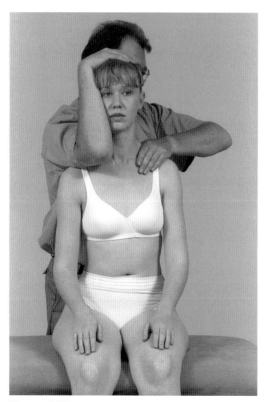

Figure 8.93

6. Positioning for thrust

Keeping your position behind the patient, place your right hand and forearm alongside the right side of the patient's head and neck and gently rest the palm of your hand over the top of the patient's head (Fig. 8.93). Ensure that your forearm remains anterior to and just over, the patient's ear. This hand will introduce and control the rotation and sidebending leverages.

Use your right hand to introduce a small amount of head and neck extension (Fig. 8.94). Now introduce cervical sidebending to the left by allowing the patient's body weight to fall slightly to the right. Keeping the patient's head centred over the sacrum, guide the neck into left sidebending with your right arm against the right side of the patient's head. A vertex compression force can be added to assist in localizing forces to the T2–3 segment. Ensure that your applicator thumb forms a straight line with your left forearm.

7. Adjustments to achieve appropriate pre-thrust tension

Ensure the patient remains relaxed. Maintaining all holds, make any necessary changes in flexion, extension, sidebending or rotation until you can sense a state of appropriate tension and leverage. The patient should not be aware of any pain or discomfort. Make these final adjustments by balancing the pressure and direction of forces

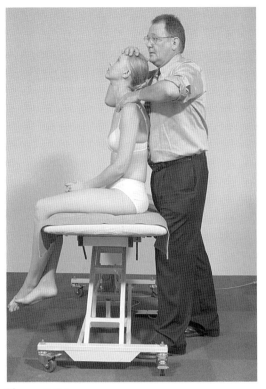

Figure 8.94

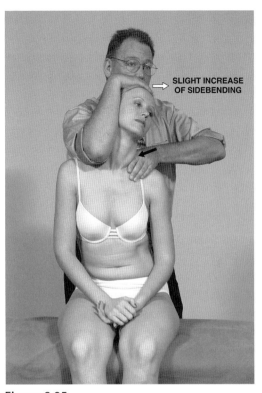

SLIGHT INCREASE
OF SIDEBENDING

Figure 8.95

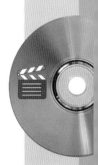

between the left hand against the contact point and the right hand and forearm against the patient's head and neck.

8. Immediately pre-thrust

Relax and adjust your balance as necessary. Keep your head up and ensure that your contacts are firm and that the patient's body weight and position are well controlled. An effective HVLA thrust technique is best achieved if the operator and patient are relaxed and not holding themselves rigid. This is a common impediment to achieving effective cavitation.

9. Delivering the thrust

This technique uses ligamentous myofascial tension locking and not facet apposition locking. This approach generally requires a greater emphasis on the exaggeration of primary leverage than is the case with facet apposition locking techniques.

Apply a HVLA thrust to the left side of the spinous process of T2 in the direction of the patient's right axilla. At the same time, increase head and neck sidebending to the left with your right arm (Fig. 8.95). The thrust on the spinous process of T2 and the increase in neck sidebending to the left focus forces at the T2–3 segment and causes cavitation at that level. The thrust is induced by a very rapid contraction of the shoulder adductors.

The thrust, although very rapid, must never be excessively forcible. The aim should be to use the absolute minimum force necessary to achieve joint cavitation. A common fault arises from the use of excessive amplitude with insufficient velocity of thrust.

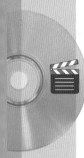

SUMMARY

Cervicothoracic spine C7–T3 Sidebending gliding

Patient sitting

Ligamentous myofascial tension locking

- **Contact point:** Left side of the T2 spinous process

- **Applicator:** Thumb of left hand

- **Patient positioning:** Patient sitting with back towards the operator

- **Operator stance:** Behind the patient

- **Palpation of contact point:** Place your left thumb against the left side of the T2 spinous process. Spread the fingers of your left hand to rest over the patient's trapezius muscle and clavicle (Fig. 8.92)

- **Positioning for thrust:** Place your right hand and forearm alongside the right side of the patient's head and neck (Fig. 8.93). Use your right hand to introduce a small amount of head and neck extension (Fig. 8.94). Introduce left sidebending to the cervical spine localizing forces to the T2–3 segment. Ensure that your applicator thumb forms a straight line with your left forearm

- **Adjustments to achieve appropriate pre-thrust tension**

- **Immediately pre-thrust:** Relax and adjust your balance

- **Delivering the thrust:** The thrust is directed towards the patient's right axilla. Simultaneously, apply a rapid increase of head and neck sidebending to the left (Fig. 8.95)

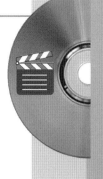

Cervicothoracic spine C7–T3
Sidebending gliding

Patient sidelying

Assume somatic dysfunction (S-T-A-R-T) is identified and you wish to use a sidebending gliding thrust, parallel to the apophysial joint plane, to produce cavitation at the T2–3 apophysial joint (Figs 8.96, 8.97).

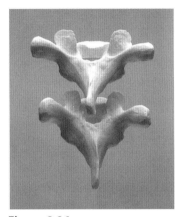

Figure 8.96

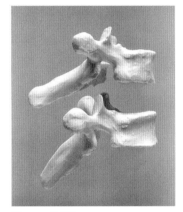

Figure 8.97

KEY

✳ Stabilization

● Applicator

→ Plane of thrust (operator)

⇨ Direction of body movement (patient)

Note: The dimensions for the arrows are not a pictorial representation of the amplitude or force of the thrust.

1. **Contact point**

Right side of the spinous process of T2.

2. **Applicator**

Thumb of left hand.

3. **Patient positioning**

Patient lying on the left side. Flex the patient's knees and hips for stability.

4. **Operator stance**

Stand facing the patient and gently place your right arm under the head, lightly spreading your fingers around the patient's occiput. The head should now be cradled in your right arm with your upper arm against the patient's

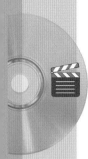

forehead and your forearm and hand supporting the head and neck.

5. **Palpation of contact point**

Locate the spinous process of T2. Place the thumb of your left hand gently but firmly against the right side of this spinous process. Spread the fingers of your left hand to enable firm contact of your thumb. This will ensure that you have good contact and will not slip off the spinous process when you apply a force against it. Maintain this contact point but do not press too hard, as it can be uncomfortable.

6. **Positioning for thrust**

Using your right arm, sidebend the patient's head and neck to the right until a sense of tension is palpable at the contact point. This sidebending is achieved by gently lifting the patient's head, within the cradle of your right arm (Fig. 8.98).

Gently introduce cervical rotation to the left until a sense of tension is palpated at the contact point (Fig. 8.99). If necessary, you may add a compression force to the patient's shoulder girdle, from your chest, to stabilize the upper torso before applying the thrust.

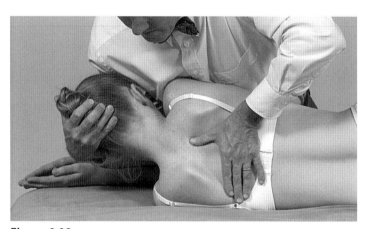

Figure 8.98

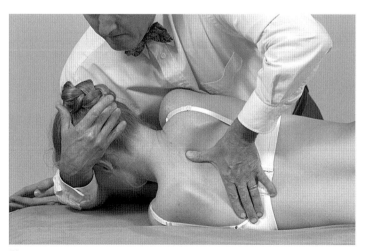

Figure 8.99

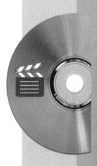

7. Adjustments to achieve appropriate pre-thrust tension

Ensure the patient remains relaxed. Maintaining all holds, make any necessary changes in flexion, extension, sidebending or rotation until you can sense a state of appropriate tension and leverage at the contact point. The patient should not be aware of any pain or discomfort. Make these final adjustments by balancing the pressure and direction of forces between the left hand against the contact point and the right hand and forearm against the patient's head and neck.

8. Immediately pre-thrust

Relax and adjust your balance as necessary. Keep your head up and ensure that your contacts are firm and that your body position is well controlled. An effective HVLA thrust technique is best achieved if the operator and patient are relaxed and not holding themselves rigid. This is a common impediment to achieving effective cavitation.

9. Delivering the thrust

Apply a HVLA thrust to the spinous process of T2 down towards the couch in the direction of the patient's left shoulder. The thrust is accompanied by a simultaneous downward application of force with your chest to the patient's right shoulder girdle. At the same time, introduce a slight increase in head and neck sidebending to the right with your right arm (Fig. 8.100). The thrust on the spinous process of T2 and slight increase in neck sidebending to the right focus forces at the T2–3 segment and causes cavitation at that level. Do not apply excessive sidebending at the time of the thrust as this can cause strain and discomfort.

The thrust, although very rapid, must never be excessively forcible. The aim should be to use the absolute minimum force necessary to achieve joint cavitation. A common fault arises from the use of excessive amplitude with insufficient velocity of thrust.

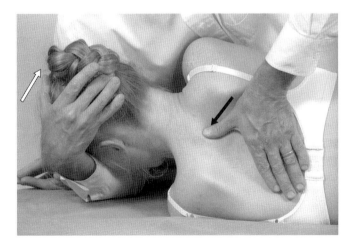

Figure 8.100

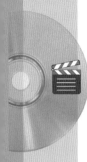

SUMMARY

Cervicothoracic spine C7–T3 Sidebending gliding

Patient sidelying

- **Contact point:** Right side of T2 spinous process

- **Applicator:** Thumb of left hand

- **Patient positioning:** Patient lying on the left side. Flex the patient's knees and hips for stability

- **Operator stance:** Facing the patient. Place your right arm under the patient's head, supporting the patient's occiput

- **Palpation of contact point:** Place the thumb of your left hand against the right side of the spinous process of T2

- **Positioning for thrust:** Using your right arm, sidebend the patient's head and neck to the right (Fig. 8.98). Introduce cervical rotation to the left until a sense of tension is palpated at the contact point (Fig. 8.99)

- **Adjustments to achieve appropriate pre-thrust tension**

- **Immediately pre-thrust:** Relax and adjust your balance

- **Delivering the thrust:** The thrust is in the direction of the patient's left shoulder and down towards the couch. The thrust is accompanied by a downward application of force with your chest to the patient's right shoulder girdle. Simultaneously, apply a slight rapid increase of head and neck sidebending to the right with your right arm (Fig. 8.100). Do not apply excessive sidebending

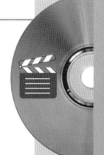

Cervicothoracic spine C7–T3
Sidebending gliding

Patient sidelying
Ligamentous myofascial tension locking

Assume somatic dysfunction (S-T-A-R-T) is identified and you wish to use a sidebending gliding thrust, parallel to the apophysial joint plane, to produce cavitation at the T2–3 apophysial joint (Figs 8.101, 8.102).

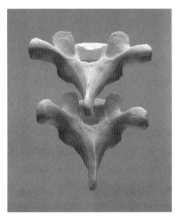

Figure 8.101

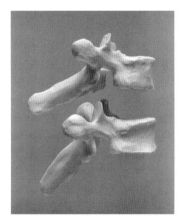

Figure 8.102

KEY

❋ Stabilization

● Applicator

→ Plane of thrust (operator)

⇨ Direction of body movement (patient)

Note: The dimensions for the arrows are not a pictorial representation of the amplitude or force of the thrust.

1. **Contact point**

Right side of the spinous process of T2.

2. **Applicator**

Thumb of left hand.

3. **Patient positioning**

Patient lying on the left side. Flex the patient's knees and hips for stability.

4. **Operator stance**

Stand facing the patient and gently place your right arm under the head, lightly spreading your fingers around the patient's occiput. The head should now be cradled in your right arm with your upper arm against the patient's

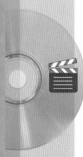

forehead and your forearm and hand supporting the head and neck.

5. Palpation of contact point

Locate the spinous process of T2. Place the thumb of your left hand gently but firmly against the right side of this spinous process. Spread the fingers of your left hand to enable firm contact of your thumb and position your left forearm over the posterior aspect of the patient's thorax and lumbar spine. This will ensure that you have good contact and will not slip off the spinous process when you apply a force against it. Maintain this contact point but do not press too hard, as it can be uncomfortable.

6. Positioning for thrust

Using your right arm, extend the patient's head and neck (Fig. 8.103). Now introduce sidebending to the right until a sense of tension is palpable at the contact point. This sidebending is achieved by gently lifting the patient's head, within the cradle of your right arm (Fig. 8.104).

If necessary, you may add a compression force to the patient's shoulder girdle, from your chest, to stabilize the upper torso before applying the thrust.

7. Adjustments to achieve appropriate pre-thrust tension

Ensure the patient remains relaxed. Maintaining all holds, make any necessary

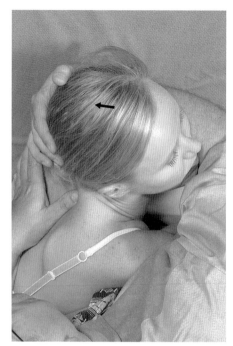

Figure 8.103

changes in flexion, extension, sidebending or rotation until you can sense a state of appropriate tension and leverage at the contact point. The patient should not be aware of any pain or discomfort. Make these final adjustments by balancing the pressure and direction of forces between the left hand against the contact point and the right hand and forearm against the patient's head and neck.

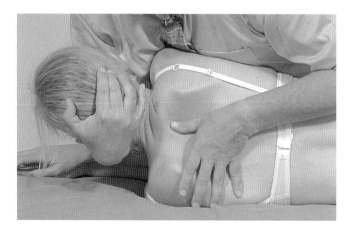

Figure 8.104

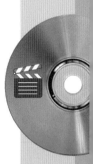

8. **Immediately pre-thrust**

Relax and adjust your balance as necessary. Keep your head up and ensure that your contacts are firm and that your body position is well controlled. An effective HVLA thrust technique is best achieved if the operator and patient are relaxed and not holding themselves rigid. This is a common impediment to achieving effective cavitation.

9. **Delivering the thrust**

This technique uses ligamentous myofascial tension locking and not facet apposition locking. This approach generally requires a greater emphasis on the exaggeration of primary leverage than is the case with facet apposition locking techniques.

Apply a HVLA thrust to the spinous process of T2 down towards the couch in the direction of the patient's left shoulder. The thrust is accompanied by a simultaneous downward application of force with your chest to the patient's right shoulder girdle. At the same time, introduce an increase in head and neck sidebending to the right with your right arm (Fig. 8.105). The thrust on the spinous process of T2 and increase in neck sidebending to the right focus forces at the T2–3 segment and causes cavitation at that level. Do not apply excessive sidebending at the time of the thrust as this can cause strain and discomfort.

The thrust, although very rapid, must never be excessively forcible. The aim should be to use the absolute minimum force necessary to achieve joint cavitation. A common fault arises from the use of excessive amplitude with insufficient velocity of thrust.

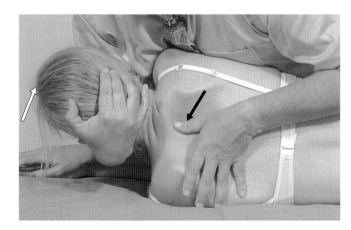

Figure 8.105

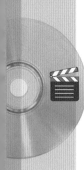

SUMMARY

Cervicothoracic spine C7–T3 Sidebending gliding

Patient sidelying

Ligamentous myofascial tension locking

- **Contact point:** Right side of T2 spinous process

- **Applicator:** Thumb of left hand

- **Patient positioning:** Patient lying on the left side. Flex the patient's knees and hips for stability

- **Operator stance:** Facing the patient. Place your right arm under the patient's head, supporting the patient's occiput

- **Palpation of contact point:** Place the thumb of your left hand against the right side of the spinous process of T2

- **Positioning for thrust:** Using your right arm, extend the patient's head and neck (Fig. 8.103). Introduce sidebending to the right until a sense of tension is palpable at the contact point (Fig. 8.104)

- **Adjustments to achieve appropriate pre-thrust tension**

- **Immediately pre-thrust:** Relax and adjust your balance

- **Delivering the thrust:** The thrust is in the direction of the patient's left shoulder and down towards the couch. The thrust is accompanied by a downward application of force with your chest to the patient's right shoulder girdle. Simultaneously, apply a rapid increase of head and neck sidebending to the right with your right arm (Fig. 8.105). Do not apply excessive sidebending

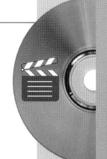

Cervicothoracic spine C7–T3
Extension gliding

Patient sitting
Ligamentous myofascial tension locking

Assume somatic dysfunction (S-T-A-R-T) is identified and you wish to use an extension gliding thrust, parallel to the apophysial joint plane, to produce joint cavitation at T2–3 (Figs 8.106, 8.107).

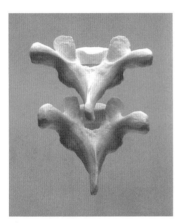

Figure 8.106

Figure 8.107

KEY

✳ Stabilization

● Applicator

→ Plane of thrust (operator)

⇨ Direction of body movement (patient)

Note: The dimensions for the arrows are not a pictorial representation of the amplitude or force of the thrust.

1. **Contact points**

(a) Spinous process of T3
(b) Patient's forearms.

2. **Applicators**

(a) Operator's sternum, with a cushion or small rolled towel, applied to the T3 spinous process (Fig. 8.108)
(b) Operator's hands applied to the patient's forearms.

3. **Patient positioning**

Sitting with arms comfortably by side.

4. **Operator stance**

Stand directly behind the patient with your feet apart and one leg behind the

173

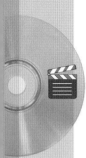

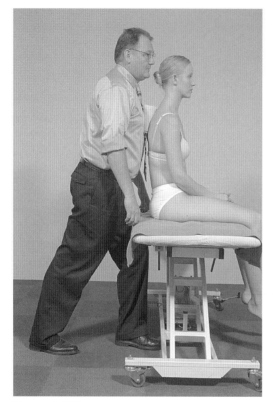

Figure 8.108

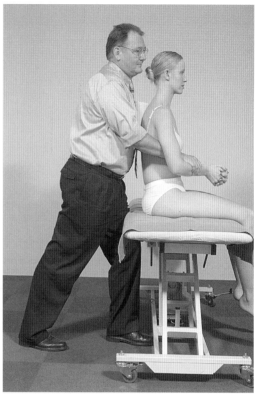

Figure 8.109

other. Bend your knees slightly to lower your body.

5. **Positioning for thrust**

Place the thrusting part of your sternum, with a cushion or small rolled towel, firmly against the spinous process of T3. Place your hands between the patient's chest and upper arms to take hold of the patients' forearms (Fig. 8.109). Maintaining your grip on the forearms ask the patient to put their hands behind their neck with fingers intertwined (Fig. 8.110). This results in your forearms contacting the patient's axillae. Lean forwards with the thrusting part of your chest against the spinous process of T3 and introduce a backwards and compressive force to the patient's arms and axillae. These combined movements introduce local extension to the thoracic spine. By balancing these different

leverages, the tension can be localized to the T2–3 segment. Maintaining all holds and pressures, bring the patient backwards until your body weight is evenly distributed between both feet.

6. **Adjustments to achieve appropriate pre-thrust tension**

Ensure your patient remains relaxed. Maintaining all holds, make any necessary changes in flexion, extension, sidebending or rotation until you can sense a state of appropriate tension and leverage at the T2–3 segment. The patient should not be aware of any pain or discomfort. Make these final adjustments by slight movements of the ankles, knees, hips and trunk. A common mistake is to lose the chest and axillae compression during the final adjustments.

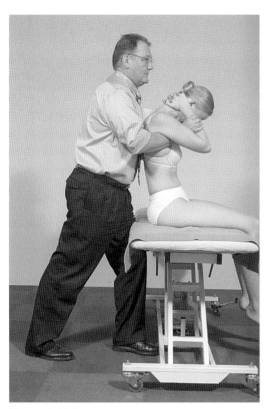

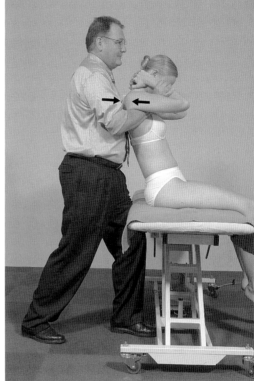

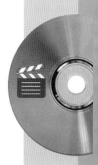

Figure 8.110

Figure 8.111

7. **Immediately pre-thrust**

Relax and adjust your balance as necessary. Keep your head up and ensure that your contacts are firm and the patient's body weight is well controlled. An effective HVLA thrust technique is best achieved if the operator and patient are relaxed and not holding themselves rigid. This is a common impediment to achieving effective cavitation.

8. **Delivering the thrust**

This technique uses ligamentous myofascial tension locking and not facet apposition locking. This approach generally requires a greater emphasis on the exaggeration of primary leverage than is the case with facet apposition locking techniques.

The shoulder girdles and thorax of the patient are now a solid mass against which a thrust may be applied. Apply a HVLA thrust towards you via your hands and forearms. Simultaneously, apply a HVLA thrust directly forwards against the spinous process of T3 via your sternum (Fig. 8.111).

The thrust, although very rapid, must never be excessively forcible. The aim should be to use the absolute minimum force necessary to achieve joint cavitation. Common faults arise from the use of excessive amplitude, insufficient velocity of thrust and lifting the patient off the couch. When delivering the thrust, particular care must be taken to not allow the patient's arms to move away from the chest wall.

This technique has some modifications:

- Respiration can be used to make the technique more effective.
- A certain degree of momentum is often necessary for success in the technique.

175

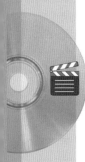

SUMMARY

Cervicothoracic spine C7–T3 Extension gliding

Patient sitting

Ligamentous myofascial tension locking

- **Contact points:**
  - Spinous process of T3
  - Patient's forearms

- **Applicators:**
  - Operator's sternum applied to the T3 spinous process (Fig. 8.108)
  - Operator's hands applied to the patient's forearms

- **Patient positioning:** Sitting with arms comfortably by side

- **Operator stance:** Directly behind the patient with your feet apart, knees bent slightly and one leg behind the other

- **Positioning for thrust:** Place your hands between the patient's chest and upper arm to take hold of the patients' forearms (Fig. 8.109). Maintaining your grip on the forearms ask the patient to put their hands behind their neck with fingers intertwined (Fig. 8.110). Lean forwards with the thrusting part of your chest against the spinous process of T3 and introduce a backwards and compressive force to the patient's arms and axillae. Maintaining all holds and pressures, bring the patient backwards until your body weight is evenly distributed between both feet

- **Adjustments to achieve appropriate pre-thrust tension**

- **Immediately pre-thrust:** Relax and adjust your balance

- **Delivering the thrust:** The direction of thrust with your arms is towards you. Simultaneously, apply a thrust directly forwards against the spinous process of T3 with your sternum (Fig. 8.111)

- **Modifications to technique:**
  - Respiration can be used to make the technique more effective
  - A certain degree of momentum is often necessary for success in the technique

Thoracic spine and rib cage

PATIENT UPPER BODY POSITIONING FOR SITTING AND SUPINE TECHNIQUES

There are a variety of upper body holds available (Figs 9.1–9.5). The hold selected for any particular technique is that which enables the operator to effectively localize forces to a specific segment of the spine or rib cage and deliver a high-velocity low-amplitude (HVLA) force in a controlled manner. Patient comfort must be a major consideration in selecting the most appropriate hold.

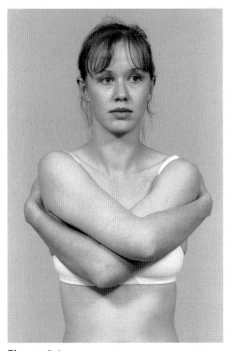

Figure 9.1

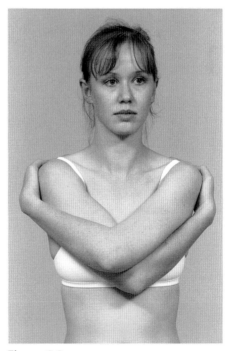

Figure 9.2

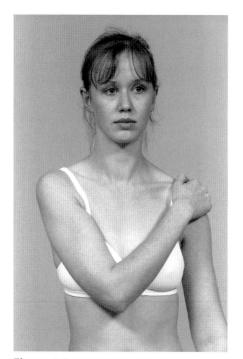

Figure 9.3

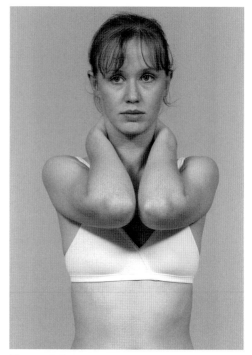

Figure 9.4

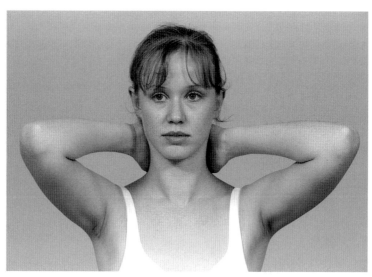

Figure 9.5

OPERATOR LOWER HAND POSITION FOR SUPINE TECHNIQUES

There are a variety of hand positions that can be adopted. The hand position selected for any particular technique is that which enables the operator to effectively localize forces to a specific segment of the spine or rib cage and deliver a HVLA force in a controlled manner.

Patient comfort must be a major consideration in selecting the most appropriate hand position.

- Neutral hand position (Fig. 9.6)
- Clenched hand position (Fig. 9.7)
- Open fist (Fig. 9.8)
- Open fist with towel (Fig. 9.9)
- Closed fist (Fig. 9.10)
- Closed fist with towel (Fig. 9.11)

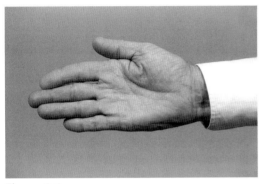

Figure 9.6

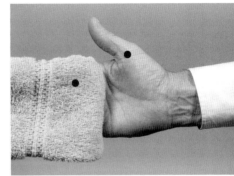

Figure 9.9

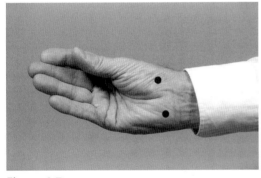

Figure 9.7

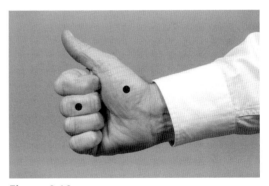

Figure 9.10

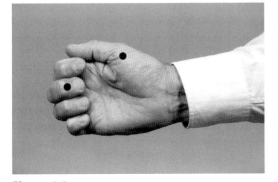

Figure 9.8

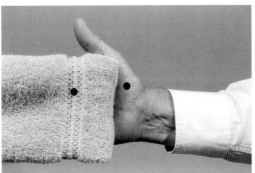

Figure 9.11

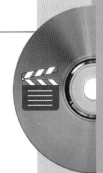

Thoracic spine T4–9
Extension gliding

Patient sitting
Ligamentous myofascial tension locking

Assume somatic dysfunction (S-T-A-R-T) is identified and you wish to use an extension gliding thrust, parallel to the apophysial joint plane, to produce joint cavitation at T5–6 (Figs 9.12, 9.13).

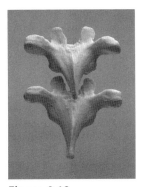

Figure 9.12

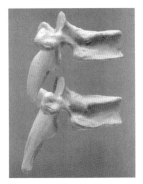

Figure 9.13

KEY

✵ Stabilization

● Applicator

→ Plane of thrust (operator)

⇨ Direction of body movement (patient)

Note: The dimensions for the arrows are not a pictorial representation of the amplitude or force of the thrust.

1. Contact points

(a) Spinous process of T6
(b) Patient's elbows.

2. Applicators

(a) Operator's sternum, with a cushion or small rolled towel, applied to the T6 spinous process (Fig. 9.14)
(b) Operator's flexed fingers, hands and wrists applied to the patient's elbows.

3. Patient positioning

Sitting with arms crossed over the chest and hands passed around the shoulders. The arms should be firmly clasped around the body as far as the patient can comfortably reach.

181

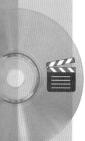

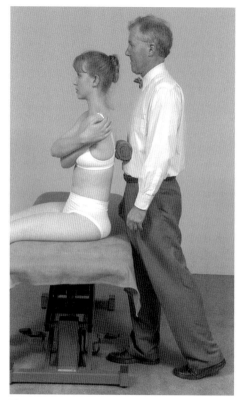

Figure 9.14

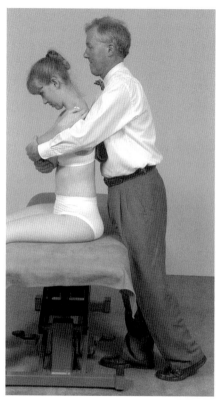

Figure 9.15

4. **Operator stance**

Stand directly behind the patient with your feet apart and one leg behind the other. Bend your knees slightly to lower your body.

5. **Positioning for thrust**

Place the thrusting part of your sternum, with a cushion or small rolled towel, firmly against the spinous process of T6. Place your hands over the patient's elbows. Lean forwards with the thrusting part of your chest against the spinous process of T6 (Fig. 9.15). Introduce a backwards (compressive) and upwards force to the patient's folded arms. These combined movements introduce local extension to the thoracic spine. By balancing these different leverages, the tension can be localized to the T5–6 segment. Maintaining all holds and pressures, bring the patient backwards until

your body weight is evenly distributed between both feet.

6. **Adjustments to achieve appropriate pre-thrust tension**

Ensure your patient remains relaxed. Maintaining all holds, make any necessary changes in flexion, extension, sidebending or rotation until you can sense a state of appropriate tension and leverage at the T5–6 segment. The patient should not be aware of any pain or discomfort. Make these final adjustments by slight movements of the ankles, knees, hips and trunk. A common mistake is to lose the chest compression during the final adjustments.

7. **Immediately pre-thrust**

Relax and adjust your balance as necessary. Keep your head up and ensure that your contacts are firm and the patient's body

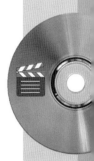

weight is well controlled. An effective HVLA thrust technique is best achieved if the operator and patient are relaxed and not holding themselves rigid. This is a common impediment to achieving effective cavitation.

8. **Delivering the thrust**

This technique uses ligamentous myofascial tension locking and not facet apposition locking. This approach generally requires a greater emphasis on the exaggeration of primary leverage than is the case with facet apposition locking techniques.

The shoulder girdles and thorax of the patient are now a solid mass against which a thrust may be applied. Apply a HVLA thrust towards you and slightly upwards in a cephalad direction via your hands. Simultaneously, apply a HVLA thrust directly forwards against the spinous process of T6 via your sternum (Fig. 9.16).

The thrust, although very rapid, must never be excessively forcible. The aim should be to use the absolute minimum force necessary to achieve joint cavitation. A common fault arises from the use of excessive amplitude with insufficient velocity of thrust.

This technique has many modifications:

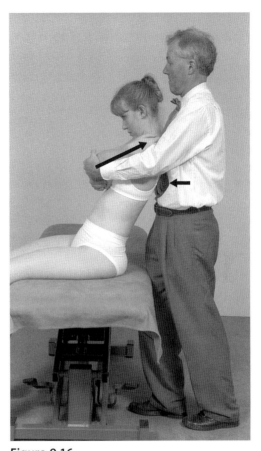

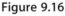

Figure 9.16

- Different shoulder girdle holds can be used
- Respiration can be used to make the technique more effective
- A certain degree of momentum is often necessary for success in the technique.

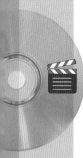

SUMMARY

Thoracic spine T4–9 Extension gliding

Patient sitting

Ligamentous myofascial tension locking

- **Contact points:**
  - Spinous process of T6
  - Patient's elbows

- **Applicators:**
  - Operator's sternum applied to the T6 spinous process (Fig. 9.14)
  - Operator's flexed fingers, hands and wrists applied to the patient's elbows

- **Patient positioning:** Sitting with arms crossed over chest

- **Operator stance:** Directly behind the patient with your feet apart, knees bent slightly and one leg behind the other

- **Positioning for thrust:** Lean forwards with the thrusting part of your chest against the spinous process of T6 (Fig. 9.15). Introduce a backwards (compressive) and upwards force to the patient's folded arms. Maintaining all holds and pressures, bring the patient backwards until your body weight is evenly distributed between both feet

- **Adjustments to achieve appropriate pre-thrust tension**

- **Immediately pre-thrust:** Relax and adjust your balance

- **Delivering the thrust:** The direction of thrust with your arms is towards you and slightly upwards. Simultaneously, apply a thrust directly forwards against the spinous process of T6 with your sternum (Fig. 9.16)

- **Modifications to technique:**
  - Different shoulder girdle holds can be used
  - Respiration can be used to make the technique more effective
  - A certain degree of momentum is often necessary for success in the technique

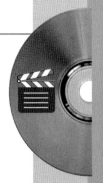

Thoracic spine T4–9
Flexion gliding

Patient supine
Ligamentous myofascial tension locking

Assume somatic dysfunction (S-T-A-R-T) is identified and you wish to use a flexion gliding thrust, parallel to the apophysial joint plane, to produce joint cavitation at T5–6 (Figs 9.17, 9.18).

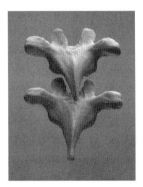

Figure 9.17

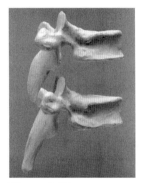

Figure 9.18

KEY

❋ Stabilization

● Applicator

→ Plane of thrust (operator)

⇨ Direction of body movement (patient)

Note: The dimensions for the arrows are not a pictorial representation of the amplitude or force of the thrust.

1. **Contact points**

(a) Transverse processes of T6
(b) Patient's elbows.

2. **Applicators**

(a) Palm of the operator's right hand, held in a clenched position
(b) Operator's lower sternum or upper abdomen.

3. **Patient positioning**

Supine with the arms crossed over the chest and hands passed around the shoulders. The arms should be firmly clasped round the body as far as the patient can comfortably reach (Fig. 9.19).

185

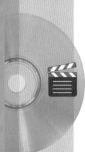

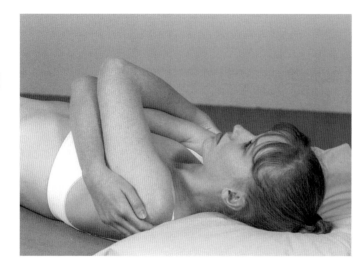

Figure 9.19

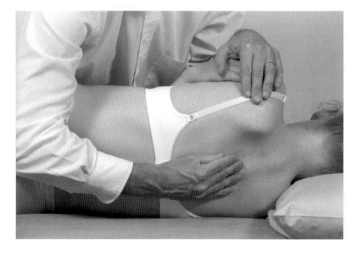

Figure 9.20

4. Operator stance

Stand on the right side of the patient, facing the head of the couch.

5. Positioning for thrust

Reach over the patient with your left hand to take hold of the left shoulder and gently pull it towards you. With your right hand, locate the transverse processes of T6. Now place the clenched palm of your right hand against the transverse processes of T6 (Fig. 9.20).

Keeping the right hand pressed against the transverse processes of T6, roll the patient back to the supine position. As the patient

approaches the supine position, transfer your left hand and forearm to support the patient's head, neck and upper thoracic spine (Fig. 9.21).

Allow the patient to roll fully into the supine position. Flex the patient's head, neck and upper thoracic spine until tension is localized to the T5–6 segment. Lean over the patient and rest your lower sternum or upper abdomen on the patient's elbows. Initially, a slow but firm pressure is applied with your lower sternum or upper abdomen downwards towards the couch. Maintaining this downward leverage,

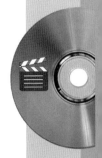

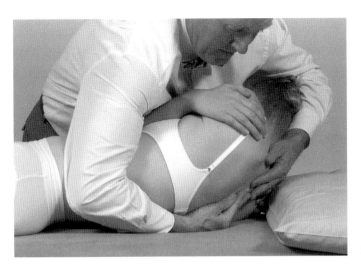

Figure 9.21

introduce a force in line with the patient's upper arms. By balancing these different leverages, tension can be localized to the T5–6 segment.

6. Adjustments to achieve appropriate pre-thrust tension

Ensure your patient remains relaxed. Maintaining all holds, make any necessary changes in flexion, extension, sidebending or rotation until you can sense a state of appropriate tension and leverage at the T5–6 segment. The patient should not be aware of any pain or discomfort. Make these final adjustments by slight movements of ankles, knees, hips and trunk. A common mistake is to lose the chest compression during the final adjustments.

7. Immediately pre-thrust

Relax and adjust your balance as necessary. Ensure that your contacts are firm and the patient's head, neck and upper thoracic spine are well controlled. An effective HVLA thrust technique is best achieved if the operator and patient are relaxed and not holding themselves rigid. This is a common impediment to achieving effective cavitation.

8. Delivering the thrust

This technique uses ligamentous myofascial tension locking and not facet apposition locking. This approach generally requires a greater emphasis on the exaggeration of primary leverage than is the case with facet apposition locking techniques.

The shoulder girdles and thorax of the patient are now a solid mass against which a thrust may be applied. Apply a HVLA thrust downwards towards the couch and in a cephalad direction via your lower sternum or upper abdomen. Simultaneously, apply a HVLA thrust with your right hand against the transverse processes in an upward and caudad direction (Fig. 9.22).

A common fault is to emphasize the thrust via the patient's shoulder girdles at the expense of the thrust against the transverse processes. The hand contacting the transverse processes of T6 must actively participate in the generation of thrust forces.

The thrust, although very rapid, must never be excessively forcible. The aim should be to use the absolute minimum force necessary to achieve joint cavitation. A common fault arises from the use of excessive amplitude with insufficient velocity of thrust.

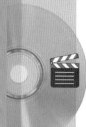

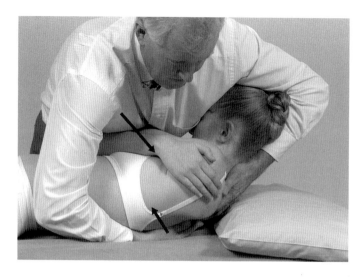

Figure 9.22

This technique has many modifications:

- Different shoulder girdle holds can be used
- Different applicators can be used
- Respiration can be used to make the technique more effective.

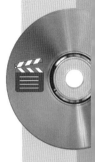

SUMMARY

Thoracic spine T4–9 Flexion gliding

Patient supine

Ligamentous myofascial tension locking

- **Contact points:**
  - Transverse processes of T6
  - Patient's elbows

- **Applicators:**
  - Palm of the operator's right hand, held in a clenched position
  - Operator's lower sternum or upper abdomen

- **Patient positioning:** Supine with arms crossed over chest (Fig. 9.19)

- **Operator stance:** To the right side of the patient, facing the couch

- **Positioning for thrust:** Take hold of the patient's left shoulder and pull it towards you. Place the clenched palm of your right hand against the transverse processes of T6 (Fig. 9.20). Roll the patient back to the supine position. As the patient approaches the supine position, transfer your left hand and forearm to support the patient's head, neck and upper thoracic spine (Fig. 9.21). Allowing the patient to roll fully into the supine position, flex the head, neck and upper thoracic spine until tension is localized to the T5–6 segment. Apply a firm pressure with your lower sternum or upper abdomen downward towards the couch. Maintaining this downward leverage, introduce a force towards the patient's head in line with the patient's upper arms

- **Adjustments to achieve appropriate pre-thrust tension**

- **Immediately pre-thrust:** Relax and adjust your balance

- **Delivering the thrust:** The direction of thrust is downwards towards the couch and in a cephalad direction via your lower sternum or upper abdomen. Simultaneously, apply a thrust with your right hand against the transverse processes in an upward and caudad direction (Fig. 9.22). The hand contacting the transverse processes of T6 must actively participate in the generation of thrust forces

- **Modifications to technique:**
  - Different shoulder girdle holds can be used
  - Different applicators can be used
  - Respiration can be used to make the technique more effective

189

Thoracic spine T4–9
Rotation gliding

Patient supine
Ligamentous myofascial tension locking

Assume somatic dysfunction (S-T-A-R-T) is identified and you wish to use a rotation gliding thrust, parallel to the apophysial joint plane, to produce joint cavitation at T5–6 (Figs 9.23, 9.24).

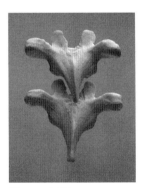

Figure 9.23

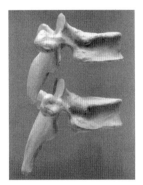

Figure 9.24

KEY

❋ Stabilization

● Applicator

→ Plane of thrust (operator)

⇨ Direction of body movement (patient)

Note: The dimensions for the arrows are not a pictorial representation of the amplitude or force of the thrust.

1. **Contact points**

(a) Left transverse process of T6
(b) Patient's elbows and left forearm.

2. **Applicators**

(a) Palm of the operator's right hand, held in a clenched position
(b) Operator's lower sternum or upper abdomen.

3. **Patient positioning**

Supine with the arms crossed over the chest and the hands passed around the shoulders. The left arm is placed over the right arm (Fig. 9.25). The arms should be firmly clasped around the body as far as the patient can comfortably reach.

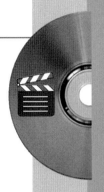

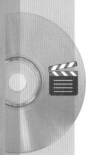

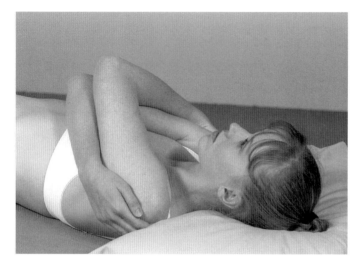

Figure 9.25

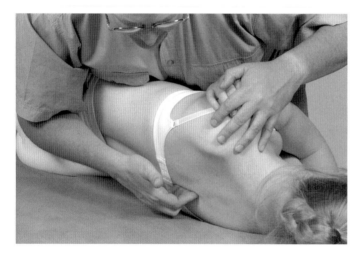

Figure 9.26

4. Operator stance

Stand on the right side of the patient, facing the couch.

5. Positioning for thrust

Reach over the patient with your left hand to take hold of the left shoulder and gently pull the patient's shoulder towards you (Fig. 9.26). With your right hand, locate the transverse processes of T6. Now place the thenar eminence of your right hand

against the left transverse process of T6 (Fig. 9.27).

Keeping contact with the left transverse process of T6, roll the patient back towards the supine position. Rest your lower sternum or upper abdomen on the patient's elbows and left forearm (Fig. 9.28).

Initially, a slow but firm pressure is applied with your lower sternum or upper abdomen downward towards the couch. Maintaining this downward leverage, introduce left rotation of the patient's upper thorax by directing forces

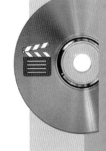

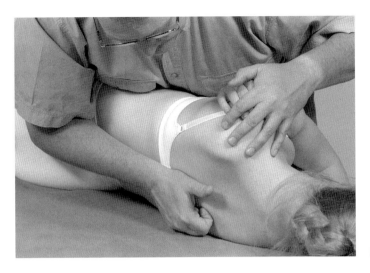

Figure 9.27

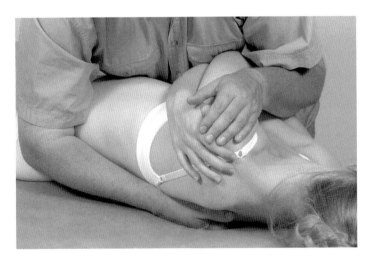

Figure 9.28

towards the patient's left shoulder along the line of the patient's left upper arm. By balancing these different leverages, tension can be localized to the T5–6 segment.

6. Adjustments to achieve appropriate pre-thrust tension

Ensure your patient remains relaxed. Maintaining all holds, make any necessary changes in flexion, extension, sidebending or rotation until you can sense a state of appropriate tension and leverage at the T5–6 segment. The patient should not be aware of any pain or discomfort. Make these final

adjustments by slight movements of the ankles, knees, hips and trunk. A common mistake is to lose the chest compression during the final adjustments.

7. Immediately pre-thrust

Relax and adjust your balance as necessary. Keep your head up and ensure that your contacts are firm and the patient's body weight is well controlled. An effective HVLA thrust technique is best achieved if the operator and patient are relaxed and not holding themselves rigid. This is a common impediment to achieving effective cavitation.

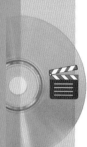

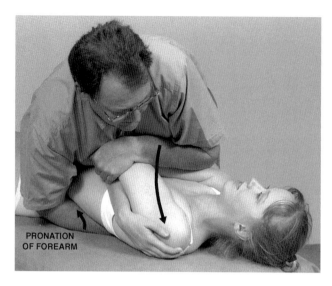

PRONATION
OF FOREARM

Figure 9.29

8. Delivering the thrust

This technique uses ligamentous myofascial tension locking and not facet apposition locking. This approach generally requires a greater emphasis on the exaggeration of primary leverage than is the case with facet apposition locking techniques.

The shoulder girdles and thorax of the patient are now a solid mass against which a thrust may be applied. Apply a HVLA thrust downwards towards the couch and in the line of the patient's left upper arm via your lower sternum or upper abdomen. Simultaneously, apply a HVLA thrust with your right thenar eminence upwards against the left transverse process of T6 (Fig. 9.29). The force is produced by rapid pronation of your right forearm.

A common fault is to emphasize the thrust via the patient's shoulder girdles at the expense of the thrust against the left transverse process. The hand contacting the transverse process of T6 must actively participate in the generation of thrust forces.

The thrust, although very rapid, must never be excessively forcible. The aim should be to use the absolute minimum force necessary to achieve joint cavitation. A common fault arises from the use of excessive amplitude with insufficient velocity of thrust.

This technique has many modifications:

- Different shoulder girdle holds can be used
- Different applicators can be used
- Respiration can be used to make the technique more effective.

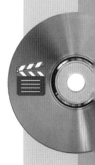

SUMMARY

Thoracic spine T4–9 Rotation gliding

Patient supine

Ligamentous myofascial tension locking

- **Contact points:**
  - Left transverse process of T6
  - Patient's elbows and left forearm

- **Applicators:**
  - Palm of the operator's right hand, held in a clenched position
  - Operator's lower sternum or upper abdomen

- **Patient positioning:** Supine with arms crossed over the chest (Fig. 9.25)

- **Operator stance:** To the right side of the patient, facing the couch

- **Positioning for thrust:** Take hold of the patient's left shoulder and pull it towards you (Fig. 9.26). Place the thenar eminence of your right hand against the left transverse process of T6 (Fig. 9.27). Roll the patient back towards the supine position. Rest your lower sternum or upper abdomen on the patient's elbows and left forearm (Fig. 9.28). Apply a slow firm pressure with your lower sternum or upper abdomen downwards towards the couch. Maintaining this downward leverage, introduce left rotation of the patient's upper thorax by directing forces towards the patient's left shoulder along the line of the patient's left upper arm

- **Adjustments to achieve appropriate pre-thrust tension**

- **Immediately pre-thrust:** Relax and adjust your balance

- **Delivering the thrust:** The direction of thrust is downwards towards the couch and in the line of the patient's left upper arm via your lower sternum or upper abdomen. Simultaneously, apply a thrust with your right thenar eminence upwards against the left transverse process of T6 (Fig. 9.29). The force is produced by rapid pronation of your right forearm. The hand contacting the transverse process of T6 must actively participate in the generation of thrust forces

- **Modifications to technique:**
  - Different shoulder girdle holds can be used
  - Different applicators can be used
  - Respiration can be used to make the technique more effective

195

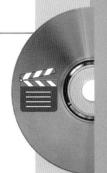

Thoracic spine T4–9
Rotation gliding

Patient prone
Short-lever technique

Assume somatic dysfunction (S-T-A-R-T) is identified and you wish to use a rotation gliding thrust, parallel to the apophysial joint plane, to produce joint cavitation at T5–6 (Figs 9.30, 9.31).

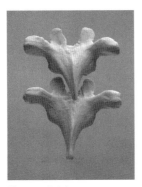

Figure 9.30

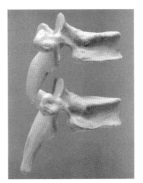

Figure 9.31

KEY

✷ Stabilization

● Applicator

→ Plane of thrust (operator)

⇨ Direction of body movement (patient)

Note: The dimensions for the arrows are not a pictorial representation of the amplitude or force of the thrust.

1. Contact points

Transverse processes of T5 (right applicator) and T6 (left applicator).

2. Applicators

Hypothenar eminence of left and right hands.

3. Patient positioning

Patient lying prone with the head and neck in a comfortable position and arms hanging over the edge of the couch.

4. Operator stance

Stand at the left side of the patient, feet spread slightly and facing the patient. Stand as erect as possible and avoid crouching as

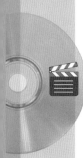

this will limit the technique and restrict delivery of the thrust.

5. Palpation of contact points

There are many different ways to perform this technique. This is one approach. Locate the transverse processes of T5 and T6. Place the hypothenar eminence of your right hand against the left transverse process of T5 and establish a firm contact (Fig. 9.32). Place the hypothenar eminence of your left hand against the right transverse process of T6 (Fig. 9.33). Ensure that you have good contact and will not slip across the skin or superficial musculature when you apply downward and caudad or

cephalad forces against the transverse processes. Maintain these contact points.

6. Positioning for thrust

This is a short-lever technique and the velocity of the thrust is critical. Move your centre of gravity over the patient by leaning your body weight forwards onto your arms and hypothenar eminences (Fig. 9.34). Shifting your centre of gravity forwards will direct a downward pressure on the transverse processes. You must apply an additional force directed caudad with the left hand and cephalad with the right hand. The final direction of thrust is influenced by the degree of

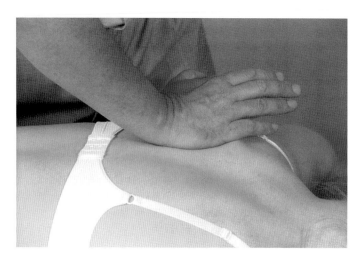

Figure 9.32

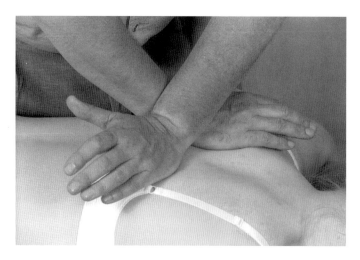

Figure 9.33

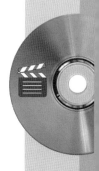

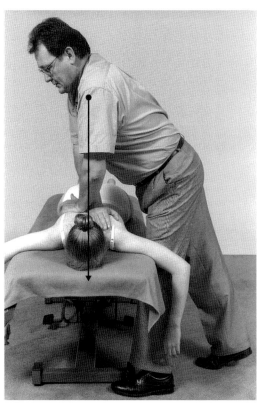

Figure 9.34

towards the end range of available joint gliding. Extensive practice is necessary to develop an appreciation of the required tension.

7. Adjustments to achieve appropriate pre-thrust tension

Ensure your patient remains relaxed. Maintaining all holds and pressure upon the transverse processes, make any necessary changes by introducing very slight components of extension, sidebending and rotation until you sense a state of appropriate tension and leverage at the T5–6 segment. The patient should not be aware of any pain or discomfort.

8. Immediately pre-thrust

Relax and adjust your balance as necessary. Keep your head up and ensure that your contacts are firm. An effective HVLA thrust technique is best achieved if the operator and patient are relaxed and not holding themselves rigid. This is a common impediment to achieving effective cavitation.

9. Delivering the thrust

Apply a HVLA thrust directed in a downward and cephalad direction against the transverse process of T5 while simultaneously applying a thrust downwards and in a caudad direction against the transverse process of T6 (Fig. 9.35).

thoracic kyphosis and any pre-existing scoliosis. This technique does not use facet apposition locking. The pre-thrust tension is achieved by positioning the T5–6 segment

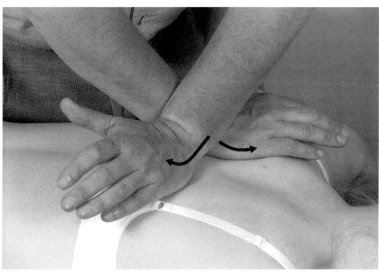

Figure 9.35

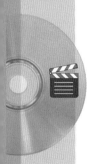

The thrust, although very rapid, must never be excessively forcible. The aim should be to use the absolute minimum force necessary to achieve joint cavitation. A common fault arises from the use of excessive amplitude with insufficient velocity of thrust.

SUMMARY

Thoracic spine T4–9 Rotation gliding

Patient prone

Short-lever technique

- **Contact points:** Transverse processes of T5 (right applicator) and T6 (left applicator)

- **Applicators:** Hypothenar eminence of left and right hands

- **Patient positioning:** Prone with arms hanging over the edge of the couch

- **Operator stance:** To the left side of the patient, facing the couch

- **Palpation of contact points:** Place the hypothenar eminence of your right hand against the left transverse process of T5 and establish a firm contact (Fig. 9.32). Place the hypothenar eminence of your left hand against the right transverse process of T6 (Fig. 9.33)

- **Positioning for thrust:** This is a short-lever technique and the velocity of the thrust is critical. Move your centre of gravity over the patient by leaning your body weight forwards onto your arms and hypothenar eminences (Fig. 9.34). Apply an additional force directed caudad with the left hand and cephalad with the right hand

- **Adjustments to achieve appropriate pre-thrust tension**

- **Immediately pre-thrust:** Relax and adjust your balance

- **Delivering the thrust:** The direction of thrust is in a downward and cephalad direction against the transverse process of T5 while simultaneously applying a thrust downwards and in a caudad direction against the transverse process of T6 (Fig. 9.35)

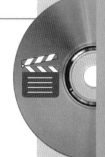

Ribs R1–3
Patient prone

Gliding thrust

Assume somatic dysfunction (S-T-A-R-T) is identified and you wish to produce cavitation at the costotransverse joint of the second rib on the right (Figs 9.36, 9.37).

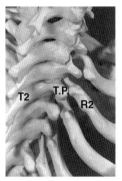

Figure 9.36

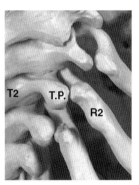

Figure 9.37

KEY

✳ Stabilization

● Applicator

→ Plane of thrust (operator)

⇨ Direction of body movement (patient)

Note: The dimensions for the arrows are not a pictorial representation of the amplitude or force of the thrust.

1. **Contact point**

Angle of the second rib on the right.

2. **Applicator**

Hypothenar eminence of the right hand.

3. **Patient positioning**

Patient prone with the point of the chin resting on the couch and the arms hanging over the edge of the couch. Introduce a small amount of sidebending to the left by gently lifting and moving the chin to the patient's left (Fig. 9.38). Do not introduce too much sidebending.

4. **Operator stance**

Head of the couch, feet spread slightly. Stand as erect as possible and avoid crouching over

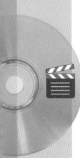

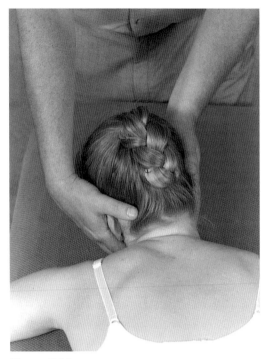

Figure 9.38

the patient as this will limit the technique and restrict delivery of the thrust.

5. **Palpation of contact point**

Locate the angle of the second rib on the right. Place the hypothenar eminence of your right hand gently, but firmly, against the rib angle. Ensure that you have good contact and will not slip across the skin or superficial musculature when you apply a caudad and downward force towards the couch against the angle of the second rib. Maintain this contact point.

6. **Positioning for thrust**

Keeping your position at the head of the couch, gently place your left hand against the right side of the patient's head and neck. While maintaining the left sidebending, introduce rotation to the right, in the cervical and upper thoracic spine, by applying gentle pressure to the right side of the patient's head and neck with your left hand (Fig. 9.39). Maintaining all holds and pressures, complete the rotation of the patient's head and neck

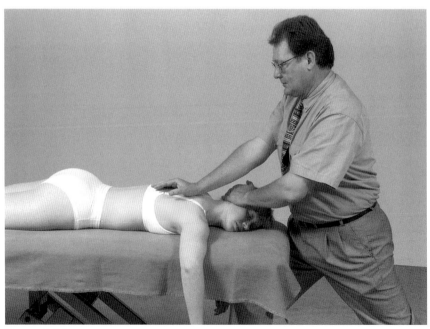

Figure 9.39

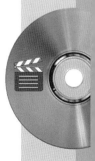

until a sense of tension is palpated at your right hypothenar eminence. Keep firm pressure against the contact point.

7. Adjustments to achieve appropriate pre-thrust tension

Ensure the patient remains relaxed. Maintaining all holds, make any necessary changes in extension, sidebending or rotation until you can sense a state of appropriate tension and leverage. The patient should not be aware of any pain or discomfort. You make these final adjustments by altering the pressure and direction of forces between the left hand against the patient's head and neck and your right hypothenar eminence against the contact point.

8. Immediately pre-thrust

Relax and adjust your balance as necessary. Keep your head up and ensure that your contacts are firm and your body position is well controlled. An effective HVLA thrust technique is best achieved if the operator and patient are relaxed and not holding

themselves rigid. This is a common impediment to achieving effective cavitation.

9. Delivering the thrust

Apply a HVLA thrust to the angle of the second rib on the right directed downwards towards the couch and also in a caudad direction towards the patient's right iliac crest. Simultaneously, apply a slight, rapid increase of head and neck rotation to the right with your left hand (Fig. 9.40). You must not overemphasize the thrust with the left hand against the patient's head and neck. Your left hand stabilizes the leverages and maintains the position of the head and cervical spine against the thrust imposed upon the contact point. The thrust is induced by a very rapid contraction of the triceps, shoulder adductors and internal rotators.

The thrust, although very rapid, must never be excessively forcible. The aim should be to use the absolute minimum force necessary to achieve joint cavitation. A common fault arises from the use of excessive amplitude with insufficient velocity of thrust.

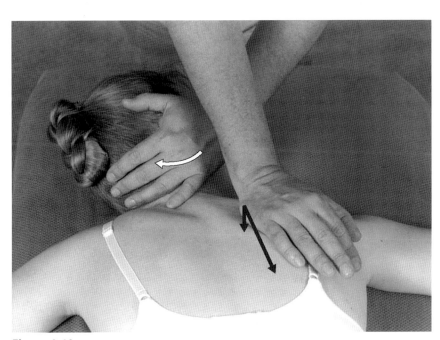

Figure 9.40

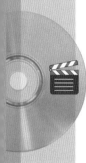

SUMMARY

Ribs R1–3 Patient prone

Gliding thrust

- **Contact point:** Angle of the right second rib

- **Applicator:** Hypothenar eminence

- **Patient positioning:** Patient prone with the chin resting on the couch and arms hanging over the edge of the couch. Introduce sidebending to the left (Fig. 9.38). Do not introduce too much sidebending

- **Operator stance:** Head of the couch, feet spread slightly

- **Palpation of contact point:** Place your hypothenar eminence against the angle of the second rib on the right. Ensure that you have good contact and will not slip across the skin or superficial musculature when you apply a caudad and downward force towards the couch against the angle of the second rib

- **Positioning for thrust:** Place your left hand against the right side of the patient's head and neck. Rotate the cervical and upper thoracic spine to the right, by applying pressure to the right side of the patient's head and neck with your left hand until a sense of tension is palpated at the contact point (Fig. 9.39)

- **Adjustments to achieve appropriate pre-thrust tension**

- **Immediately pre-thrust:** Relax and adjust your balance

- **Delivering the thrust:** The thrust to the angle of the second rib on the right is directed downwards towards the couch and also in a caudad direction towards the patient's right iliac crest. Simultaneously, apply a slight, rapid increase of head and neck rotation to the right with your left hand (Fig. 9.40). You must not overemphasize the thrust with the left hand against the patient's head and neck

9.6

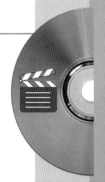

Ribs R4–10
Patient supine

Gliding thrust
Ligamentous myofascial tension locking

Assume somatic dysfunction (S-T-A-R-T) is identified and you wish to produce cavitation at the costotransverse joint of the sixth rib on the left (Fig. 9.41).

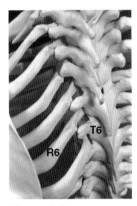

Figure 9.41

KEY

✳ Stabilization

● Applicator

➜ Plane of thrust (operator)

⇨ Direction of body movement (patient)

Note: The dimensions for the arrows are not a pictorial representation of the amplitude or force of the thrust.

1. **Contact points**

(a) Sixth rib on the left, just lateral to the transverse process of T6
(b) Patient's elbows and left forearm.

2. **Applicators**

(a) Hypothenar eminence of the operator's right hand
(b) Operator's lower sternum or upper abdomen.

3. **Patient positioning**

Supine with the arms crossed over the chest and the hands passed around the shoulders. The left arm is placed over the right arm. The arms should be firmly clasped around the body as far as the patient can comfortably reach.

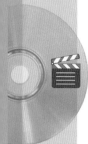

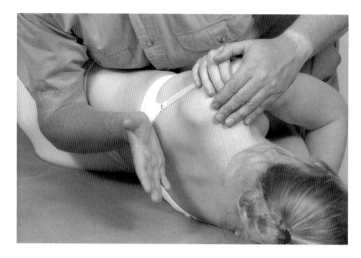

Figure 9.42

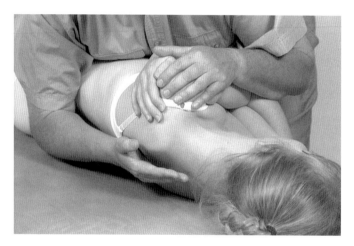

Figure 9.43

4. **Operator stance**

Stand on the right side of the patient, facing the couch.

5. **Positioning for thrust**

Reach over the patient with your left hand to take hold of the left shoulder and gently pull it towards you. With your right hand, locate the sixth rib on the left. Now place the hypothenar eminence of your right hand against the rib just lateral to the transverse process of T6 (Fig. 9.42).

Keeping contact with the rib, begin rolling the patient back to the supine position (Fig. 9.43). Continue until the

patient's elbows are directly over your hypothenar eminence. This introduces additional rotation, which is a critical element in the technique.

Rest your lower sternum or upper abdomen on the patient's elbows and left forearm. Initially, a slow but firm pressure is applied with your lower sternum or upper abdomen downwards towards the couch. Maintaining this downward leverage, introduce left rotation of the patient's upper thorax by directing forces towards the patient's left shoulder along the line of the patient's left upper arm. By balancing these different leverages, tension can be localized to the costotransverse joint of the sixth rib.

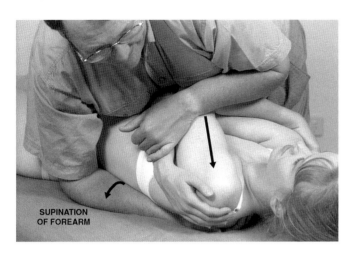

SUPINATION OF FOREARM

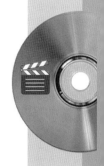

Figure 9.44

6. Adjustments to achieve appropriate pre-thrust tension

Ensure your patient remains relaxed. Maintaining all holds, make any necessary changes in flexion, extension, sidebending and rotation until you can sense a state of appropriate tension and leverage at the costotransverse joint of the sixth rib. The patient should not be aware of any pain or discomfort. Make these final adjustments by slight movements of the ankles, knees, hips and trunk. A common mistake is to lose the chest compression during the final adjustments.

7. Immediately pre-thrust

Relax and adjust your balance as necessary. Keep your head up and ensure that your contacts are firm and the patient's body weight is well controlled. An effective HVLA thrust technique is best achieved if the operator and patient are relaxed and not holding themselves rigid. This is a common impediment to achieving effective cavitation.

8. Delivering the thrust

This technique uses ligamentous myofascial tension locking and not facet apposition locking. This approach generally requires a greater emphasis on the exaggeration of primary leverage than is the case with facet apposition locking techniques.

The shoulder girdles and thorax of the patient are now a solid mass against which a thrust may be applied. Apply a HVLA thrust downward towards the couch and in the line of the patient's left upper arm via your lower sternum or upper abdomen. Simultaneously, apply a HVLA thrust with your right hypothenar eminence upward against the sixth rib (Fig. 9.44). The force is produced by rapid supination of your right forearm.

A common fault is to emphasize the thrust via the patient's shoulder girdles at the expense of the thrust against the sixth rib. The hand contacting the rib must actively participate in the generation of thrust forces.

The thrust, although very rapid, must never be excessively forcible. The aim should be to use the absolute minimum force necessary to achieve joint cavitation. A common fault arises from the use of excessive amplitude with insufficient velocity of thrust.

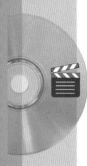

SUMMARY

Ribs R4–10 Patient supine

Gliding thrust

Ligamentous myofascial tension locking

- **Contact points:**
  - Sixth rib on the left, lateral to the transverse process
  - Patient's elbows and left forearm

- **Applicators:**
  - Hypothenar eminence of the operator's right hand
  - Operator's lower sternum or upper abdomen

- **Patient positioning:** Supine with arms crossed over the chest

- **Operator stance:** To the right side of the patient, facing the couch

- **Positioning for thrust:** Take hold of the patient's left shoulder and pull it towards you. Place the hypothenar eminence of your right hand against the rib just lateral to the left transverse process of T6 (Fig. 9.42). Roll the patient back to the supine position (Fig. 9.43). Continue until the patient's elbows are directly over your hypothenar eminence. This is a critical element in the technique. Rest your lower sternum or upper abdomen on the patient's elbows and left forearm. Apply a slow firm pressure with your lower sternum or upper abdomen downwards towards the couch. Maintaining this downward leverage, introduce left rotation of the patient's upper thorax by directing forces towards the patient's left shoulder along the line of the patient's left upper arm

- **Adjustments to achieve appropriate pre-thrust tension**

- **Immediately pre-thrust:** Relax and adjust your balance

- **Delivering the thrust:** The direction of thrust is downwards towards the couch and in the line of the patient's left upper arm via your lower sternum or upper abdomen. Simultaneously, apply a thrust with your right hypothenar eminence upwards against the sixth rib (Fig. 9.44). The force is produced by rapid supination of your right forearm. The hand contacting the rib must actively participate in the generation of thrust forces

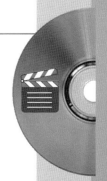

Ribs R4–10
Patient prone

Gliding thrust
Short-lever technique

Assume somatic dysfunction (S-T-A-R-T) is identified and you wish to produce cavitation at the costotransverse joint of the sixth rib on the left (Fig. 9.45).

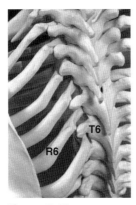

Figure 9.45

KEY

✳ Stabilization

● Applicator

→ Plane of thrust (operator)

⇨ Direction of body movement (patient)

Note: The dimensions for the arrows are not a pictorial representation of the amplitude or force of the thrust.

1. **Contact points**

Angle of left sixth rib (right applicator). Right transverse process of T6 (left applicator).

2. **Applicators**

Hypothenar eminence of left and right hands.

3. **Patient positioning**

Patient lying prone with the head and neck in a comfortable position and the arms hanging over the edge of the couch.

4. **Operator stance**

Stand at the left side of the patient, feet spread slightly and facing the patient. Stand as erect as possible and avoid crouching as this will limit

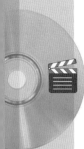

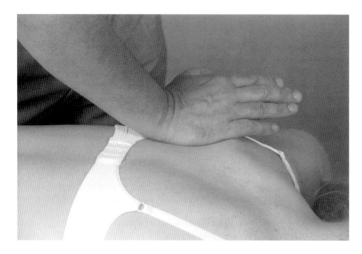

Figure 9.46

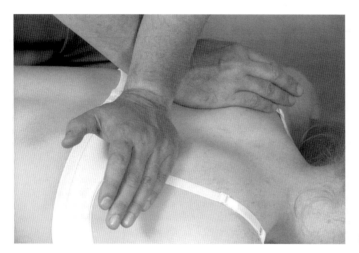

Figure 9.47

the technique and restrict delivery of the thrust.

5. Palpation of contact points

There are many different ways to perform this technique. This is one approach. Locate the transverse processes of T6. Place the hypothenar eminence of your right hand against the angle of the patient's left sixth rib and establish a firm contact (Fig. 9.46). Place the hypothenar eminence of your left hand against the right transverse process of T6 (Fig. 9.47). Ensure that you have good contact and will not slip across the skin or superficial musculature.

6. Positioning for thrust

This is a short-lever technique and as a consequence the velocity of the thrust is critical. Move your centre of gravity over the patient by leaning your body weight forwards onto your arms and hypothenar eminences (Fig. 9.48). Shifting your centre of gravity forwards will direct a downward pressure on both the transverse process of T6 and the sixth rib. You must apply an additional force directed cephalad with the right hand against the angle of the sixth rib. The final direction of thrust is influenced by the degree of thoracic kyphosis and any pre-existing scoliosis. This technique does not use facet apposition

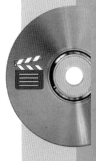

locking. The pre-thrust tension is achieved by positioning the costotransverse joint of the sixth rib towards the end range of available joint gliding. Extensive practice is necessary to develop an appreciation of the required tension.

7. Adjustments to achieve appropriate pre-thrust tension

Ensure your patient remains relaxed. Maintaining all holds, make any necessary changes in extension, sidebending and rotation until you sense a state of appropriate tension and leverage at the costotransverse joint of the sixth rib. The patient should not be aware of any pain or discomfort.

8. Immediately pre-thrust

Relax and adjust your balance as necessary. Keep your head up and ensure that your contacts are firm. An effective HVLA thrust technique is best achieved if the operator and patient are relaxed and not holding themselves rigid. This is a common impediment to achieving effective cavitation.

9. Delivering the thrust

Apply a HVLA thrust directed in a downward and cephalad direction against the angle of the sixth rib. It is important to achieve fixation of T6 by maintaining a firm downward pressure against the transverse process of T6 on the right. The thrust is generated by your right hand in contact with the sixth rib (Fig. 9.49).

The thrust, although very rapid, must never be excessively forcible. The aim should be to use the absolute minimum force necessary to achieve joint cavitation. A common fault arises from the use of excessive amplitude with insufficient velocity of thrust.

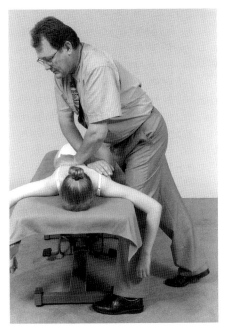

Figure 9.48

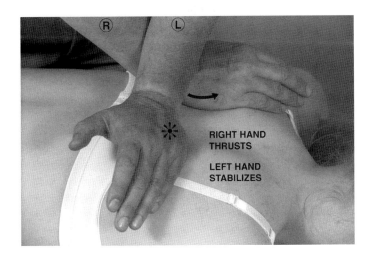

RIGHT HAND
THRUSTS

LEFT HAND
STABILIZES

Figure 9.49

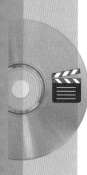

SUMMARY

Ribs R4–10 Patient prone

Gliding thrust

Short-lever technique

- **Contact points:** Angle of left sixth rib (right applicator). Right transverse process of T6 (left applicator)

- **Applicators:** Hypothenar eminence of left and right hands

- **Patient positioning:** Prone with arms hanging over the edge of the couch

- **Operator stance:** To the left side of the patient, facing the couch

- **Palpation of contact points:** Place the hypothenar eminence of your right hand against the angle of the patient's left sixth rib and establish a firm contact (Fig. 9.46). Place the hypothenar eminence of left hand against the right transverse process of T6 (Fig. 9.47)

- **Positioning for thrust:** This is a short-lever technique and the velocity of the thrust is critical. Move your centre of gravity over the patient by leaning your body weight forwards onto your arms and hypothenar eminences (Fig. 9.48). Apply an additional force directed cephalad with the right hand against the angle of the sixth rib

- **Adjustments to achieve appropriate pre-thrust tension**

- **Immediately pre-thrust:** Relax and adjust your balance

- **Delivering the thrust:** The direction of thrust is in a downward and cephalad direction against the angle of the sixth rib. It is important to achieve fixation of T6 by maintaining a firm downward pressure against the transverse process of T6 on the right. The thrust is generated by your right hand in contact with the sixth rib (Fig. 9.49)

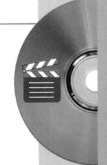

Ribs R4–10
Patient sitting

Gliding thrust
Ligamentous myofascial tension locking

Assume somatic dysfunction (S-T-A-R-T) is identified and you wish to produce cavitation at the costotransverse joint of the right sixth rib (Fig. 9.50).

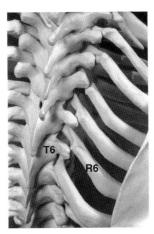

T6

R6

Figure 9.50

KEY

✳ Stabilization

● Applicator

→ Plane of thrust (operator)

⇨ Direction of body movement (patient)

Note: The dimensions for the arrows are not a pictorial representation of the amplitude or force of the thrust.

1. Contact point

Angle of right sixth rib.

2. Applicator

Hypothenar eminence of right hand.

3. Patient positioning

Sitting astride the treatment couch with the arms crossed over the chest and the hands passed around the shoulders. The arms should be firmly clasped around the body as far as the patient can comfortably reach.

4. Operator stance

Stand behind and slightly to the left of the patient with your feet spread. Pass your left

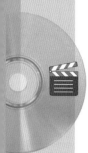

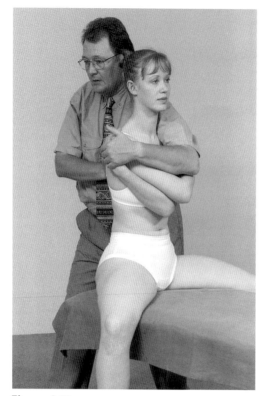

Figure 9.51

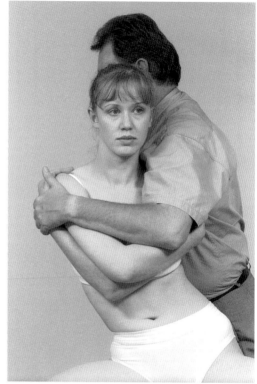

Figure 9.52

arm across the front of the patient's chest to lightly grip over the patient's right shoulder region (Fig. 9.51).

5. Positioning for thrust

Translate the patient's trunk to the right and away from you. This opens up the intercostal space between the sixth and seventh ribs (Fig. 9.52) and allows better access to the inferior aspect of the sixth rib. Place your right hypothenar eminence on the inferior surface of the angle of the sixth rib. The thorax is now rotated to the left (Fig. 9.53). Sidebending to the right is introduced to localize tension at the costotransverse joint of the sixth rib. The operator maintains as erect a posture as possible. Keep your right hypothenar eminence firmly applied to the sixth rib with your right elbow held close to your body (Fig. 9.54).

214

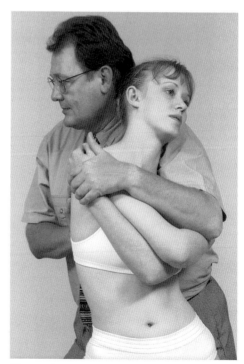

Figure 9.53

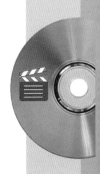

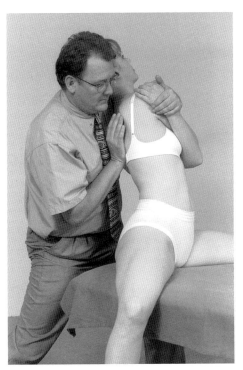

Figure 9.54

8. Delivering the thrust

This technique uses ligamentous myofascial tension locking and not facet apposition locking. This approach generally requires a greater emphasis on the exaggeration of primary leverage than is the case with facet apposition locking techniques.

A degree of momentum is necessary to achieve a successful cavitation. Rock the patient into and out of rotation while maintaining the other leverages. When you sense a state of appropriate tension and leverage at the sixth rib, apply a HVLA thrust against the inferior aspect of the angle of the rib in a cephalad and anterior direction. Simultaneously, apply slight exaggeration of left trunk rotation (Fig. 9.55).

The thrust, although very rapid, must never be excessively forcible. The aim should be to use the absolute minimum force necessary to achieve joint cavitation. A common fault arises from the use of excessive amplitude with insufficient velocity of thrust.

6. Adjustments to achieve appropriate pre-thrust tension

Ensure your patient remains relaxed. Maintaining all holds, make any necessary changes in flexion, extension, sidebending or rotation until you can sense a state of appropriate tension and leverage at the costotransverse joint of the sixth rib on the right. The patient should not be aware of any pain or discomfort. Make these final adjustments by slight movements of the shoulders, trunk, ankles, knees and hips.

7. Immediately pre-thrust

Relax and adjust your balance as necessary. An effective HVLA thrust technique is best achieved if both the operator and patient are relaxed and not holding themselves rigid. This is a common impediment to achieving effective cavitation.

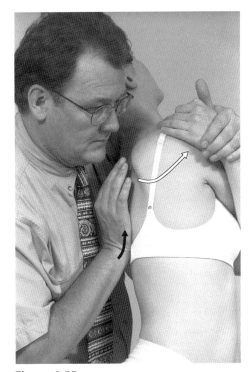

Figure 9.55

215

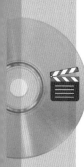

SUMMARY

Ribs R4–10 Patient sitting

Gliding thrust

Ligamentous myofascial tension locking

- **Contact point:** Angle of right sixth rib

- **Applicator:** Hypothenar eminence of right hand

- **Patient positioning:** Sitting astride the couch with the arms crossed over the chest and the hands passed around the shoulders

- **Operator stance:** Behind and slightly to the left of the patient with the feet spread. Pass your left arm across the front of the patient's chest to lightly grip over the patient's right shoulder region (Fig. 9.51)

- **Positioning for thrust:** Translate the patient's trunk to the right and away from you (Fig. 9.52). Place your right hypothenar eminence on the inferior surface of the angle of the sixth rib. The thorax is now rotated to the left (Fig. 9.53). Sidebending to the right is introduced to localize tension at the costotransverse joint of the sixth rib. The operator maintains as erect a posture as possible. Keep your right hypothenar eminence firmly applied to the sixth rib with your right elbow held close to your body (Fig. 9.54)

- **Adjustments to achieve appropriate pre-thrust tension**

- **Immediately pre-thrust:** Relax and adjust your balance

- **Delivering the thrust:** A degree of momentum is necessary to achieve a successful cavitation. The direction of thrust is in a cephalad and anterior direction against the inferior aspect of the angle of the rib. Simultaneously, apply slight exaggeration of left trunk rotation (Fig. 9.55)

Lumbar and thoracolumbar spine

UPPER BODY HOLDS FOR SIDELYING TECHNIQUES

All techniques in this manual are described with the operator taking up the axillary hold (Fig. 10.1). The hold selected for any particular technique is that which enables the operator to effectively localize forces to a specific segment of the spine and deliver a high-velocity low-amplitude (HVLA) force in a controlled manner. Patient comfort must be a major consideration in selecting the most appropriate hold.

Three alternative upper body holds are available:

- Pectoral hold (Fig. 10.2)
- Elbow hold (Fig. 10.3)
- Upper arm hold (Fig. 10.4).

LOWER BODY HOLDS FOR SIDELYING TECHNIQUES

There are a variety of lower body holds available (Figs. 10.5–10.9). The hold selected for any particular technique is that which enables the operator to effectively localize forces to a specific segment of the spine and deliver a HVLA force in a controlled manner. Patient comfort must be a major consideration in selecting the most appropriate hold.

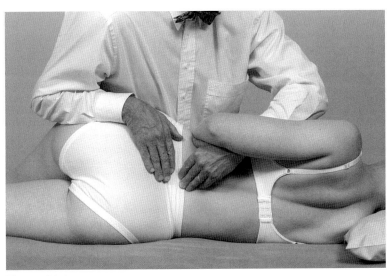

Figure 10.1

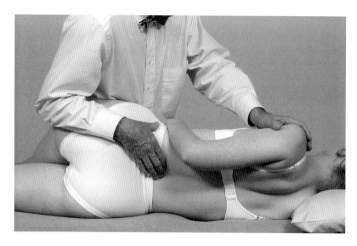

Figure 10.2

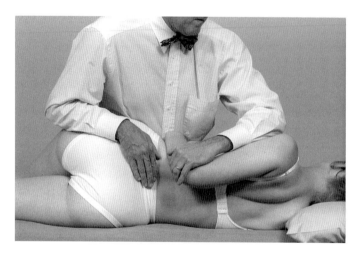

Figure 10.3

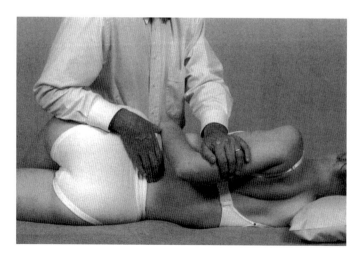

Figure 10.4

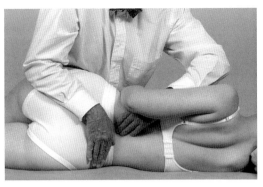

Figure 10.5

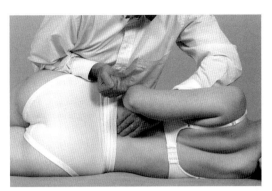

Figure 10.8

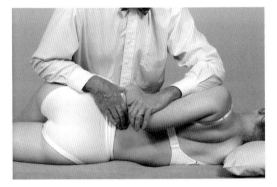

Figure 10.6

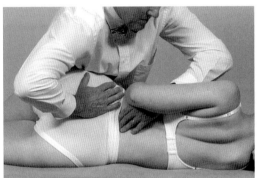

Figure 10.9

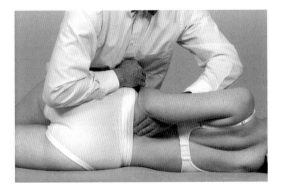

Figure 10.7

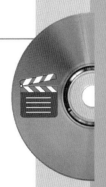

Thoracolumbar spine T10–L2
Neutral positioning

Patient sidelying
Rotation gliding thrust

Assume somatic dysfunction (S-T-A-R-T) is identified and you wish to use a rotation gliding thrust to produce cavitation at T12–L1 on the left (Figs 10.10, 10.11).

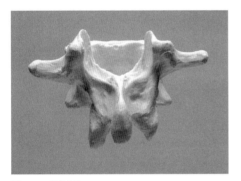

Figure 10.10

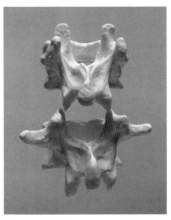

Figure 10.11

KEY

❋ Stabilization

● Applicator

➜ Plane of thrust (operator)

⇨ Direction of body movement (patient)

Note: The dimensions for the arrows are not a pictorial representation of the amplitude or force of the thrust.

1. Patient positioning

Lying on the right side with a pillow to support the head and neck. The upper portion of the couch is raised 10–15° to introduce left sidebending in the lower thoracic and upper lumbar spine. Experienced practitioners may choose to achieve the left sidebending without raising the upper portion of the couch.

Lower body. Straighten the patient's lower (right) leg and ensure that the leg and spine are in a straight line, in a neutral position. Flex the patient's upper hip and knee slightly and place the upper leg just anterior to the lower leg. The lower leg and spine should form as near a straight line as possible, with no flexion at the lower hip or knee.

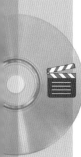

Upper body. Gently extend the patient's upper shoulder and place the patient's left forearm on the lower ribs. Using your right hand to palpate the T12–L1 interspinous space, introduce left rotation of the patient's upper body down to the T12–L1 segment. This is achieved by gently holding the patient's right elbow with your left hand and pulling it towards you, but also in a cephalad direction towards the head end of the couch. Be careful not to introduce any flexion to the spine during this movement. Left rotation is continued until your palpating hand at the T12–L1 segment begins to sense motion. Take up the axillary hold. This arm controls the upper body rotation.

2. Operator stance

Stand close to the couch with your feet spread and one leg behind the other (Fig. 10.12). Maintain an upright posture, facing slightly in the direction of the patient's upper body. Keep your right arm as close to your body as possible.

3. Positioning for thrust

Apply your right forearm to the region between gluteus medius and maximus. Your right forearm now controls lower body rotation. Your left forearm should be resting against the patient's upper pectoral and rib cage region and will control upper body rotation. First, rotate the patient's pelvis and lumbar spine towards you until motion is palpated at the T12–L1 segment. Rotate the patient's upper body away from you using your left arm until a sense of tension is palpated at the T12–L1 segment. Be careful to avoid undue pressure in the axilla. Finally, roll the patient about 10–15° towards you while maintaining the build-up of leverages at the T12–L1 segment.

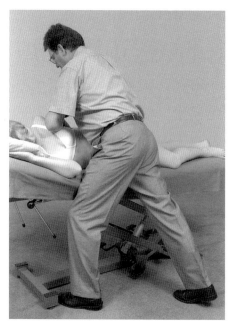

Figure 10.12

4. Adjustments to achieve appropriate pre-thrust tension

Ensure your patient remains relaxed. Maintaining all holds, make any necessary changes in flexion, extension, sidebending or rotation until you can sense a state of appropriate tension and leverage at the T12–L1 segment. The patient should not be aware of any pain or discomfort. Make these final adjustments by slight movements of the shoulders, trunk, ankles, knees and hips.

5. Immediately pre-thrust

Relax and adjust your balance as necessary. Keep your head up; looking down impedes the thrust. An effective HVLA thrust technique is best achieved if both the operator and patient are relaxed and not holding themselves rigid. This is a common impediment to achieving effective cavitation.

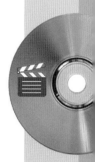

6. **Delivering the thrust**

Your left arm against the patient's pectoral region does not apply a thrust but acts as a stabilizer only. Keep the thrusting (right) arm as close to your body as possible. Apply a HVLA thrust with your right forearm against the patient's buttock. The direction of force is down towards the couch accompanied by a slight exaggeration of pelvic rotation towards the operator (Fig. 10.13).

The thrust, although very rapid, must never be excessively forcible. The aim should be to use the absolute minimum force necessary to achieve joint cavitation. A common fault arises from the use of excessive amplitude with insufficient velocity of thrust.

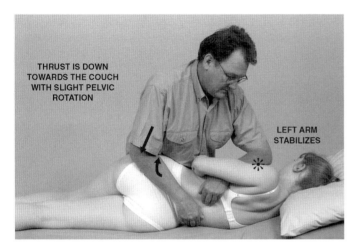

THRUST IS DOWN
TOWARDS THE COUCH
WITH SLIGHT PELVIC
ROTATION

LEFT ARM
STABILIZES

Figure 10.13

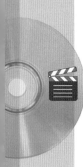

SUMMARY

Thoracolumbar spine T10–L2 Neutral positioning

Patient sidelying

Rotation gliding thrust

- **Patient positioning:** Right sidelying with the upper portion of the couch raised 10–15° to introduce left sidebending in the lower thoracic and upper lumbar spine:

  Lower body. Right leg and spine in a straight line. Left hip and knee flexed slightly and placed just anterior to the lower leg

  Upper body. Introduce left rotation of the patient's upper body until your palpating hand at T12–L1 begins to sense motion. Do not introduce any flexion to the spine during this movement. Take up the axillary hold

- **Operator stance:** Stand close to the couch, feet spread and one leg behind the other. Maintain an upright posture, facing slightly in the direction of the patient's upper body (Fig. 10.12)

- **Positioning for thrust:** Place your right forearm in the region between gluteus medius and maximus. Rotate the patient's pelvis and lumbar spine towards you until motion is palpated at the T12–L1 segment. Rotate the patient's upper body away from you until a sense of tension is palpated at the T12–L1 segment. Roll the patient about 10–15° towards you

- **Adjustments to achieve appropriate pre-thrust tension**

- **Immediately pre-thrust:** Relax and adjust your balance

- **Delivering the thrust:** The direction of thrust is down towards the couch accompanied by exaggeration of pelvic rotation towards the operator (Fig. 10.13). Your left arm against the patient's axillary region does not apply a thrust but acts as a stabilizer only

10.2

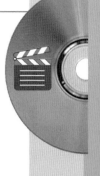

Thoracolumbar spine T10–L2
Flexion positioning

Patient sidelying
Rotation gliding thrust

Assume somatic dysfunction (S-T-A-R-T) is identified and you wish to use a rotation gliding thrust to produce cavitation at T12–L1 on the left (Figs 10.14, 10.15).

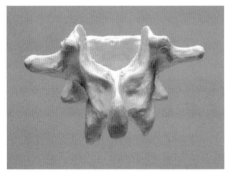

Figure 10.14

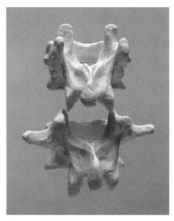

Figure 10.15

KEY

❊ Stabilization

● Applicator

→ Plane of thrust (operator)

⇨ Direction of body movement (patient)

Note: The dimensions for the arrows are not a pictorial representation of the amplitude or force of the thrust.

1. **Patient positioning**

Lying on the left side with a pillow to support the head and neck. A small pillow, or rolled towel, should be placed under the patient's waist to introduce left sidebending in the thoracolumbar spine. Experienced practitioners may choose to achieve the left sidebending without the use of a small pillow or rolled towel.

Lower body. Straighten the patient's lower (left) leg at the knee joint while keeping the left hip flexed. Flex the patient's upper hip and knee. Rest the upper flexed knee upon the edge of the couch, anterior to the left thigh, and place the patient's right foot behind the left calf. This position provides stability to the lower body.

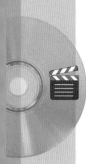

Upper body. Gently extend the patient's upper shoulder and place the patient's right forearm on the lower ribs. Using your left hand to palpate the T12–L1 interspinous space, introduce right rotation of the patient's upper body down to the T12–L1 segment. Rotation with flexion positioning is achieved by gently holding the patient's left elbow with your right hand and pulling it towards you, but also in a caudad direction towards the foot end of the couch. Left rotation is continued until your palpating hand at the T12–L1 segment begins to sense motion. Take up the axillary hold. This arm controls the upper body rotation.

2. Operator stance

Stand close to the couch with your feet spread and one leg behind the other. Maintain an upright posture, facing slightly in the direction of the patient's upper body. Keep your left arm as close to your body as possible.

3. Positioning for thrust

Apply the palmar aspect of your left forearm to the sacrum and posterior superior iliac spine. Your left forearm now controls lower body rotation. Your right forearm should be resting against the patient's upper pectoral and rib cage region and will control upper body rotation. First, rotate the patient's pelvis and lumbar spine towards you until motion is palpated at the T12–L1 segment. Rotate the patient's upper body away from you using your right arm until a sense of tension is palpated at the T12–L1 segment. Be careful to avoid undue pressure in the axilla. Finally, roll the patient about 10–15° towards you while maintaining the build-up of leverages at the T12–L1 segment.

4. Adjustments to achieve appropriate pre-thrust tension

Ensure your patient remains relaxed. Maintaining all holds, make any necessary changes in flexion, extension, sidebending or rotation until you can sense a state of appropriate tension and leverage at the T12–L1 segment. The patient should not be aware of any pain or discomfort. Make these final adjustments by slight movements of the shoulders, trunk, ankles, knees and hips.

5. Immediately pre-thrust

Relax and adjust your balance as necessary. Keep your head up; looking down impedes the thrust. An effective HVLA thrust technique is best achieved if both the operator and patient are relaxed and not holding themselves rigid. This is a common impediment to achieving effective cavitation.

6. Delivering the thrust

Your right arm against the patient's pectoral region does not apply a thrust but acts as a stabilizer only. Keep the thrusting (left) arm as close to your body as possible. Apply a HVLA thrust with your left forearm against the patient's sacrum and posterior superior iliac spine. The direction of force is down towards the couch accompanied by slight exaggeration of pelvic rotation towards the operator (Fig. 10.16).

The thrust, although very rapid, must never be excessively forcible. The aim should be to use the absolute minimum force necessary to achieve joint cavitation. A common fault arises from the use of excessive amplitude with insufficient velocity of thrust.

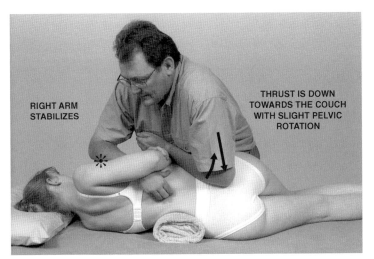

Figure 10.16

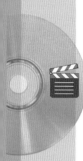

SUMMARY

Thoracolumbar spine T10–L2 Flexion positioning

Patient sidelying

Rotation gliding thrust

- **Patient positioning:** Left sidelying with a small pillow or rolled towel placed under the patient's waist to introduce left sidebending in the thoracolumbar spine:

  Lower body. Left hip flexed with knee extended. Right hip and knee flexed with patient's right foot behind the left calf

  Upper body. Introduce right rotation of the patient's upper body until your palpating hand at T12–L1 begins to sense motion. Introduce flexion to the spine during this movement. Take up the axillary hold

- **Operator stance:** Stand close to the couch, feet spread and one leg behind the other. Maintain an upright posture, facing slightly in the direction of the patient's upper body

- **Positioning for thrust:** Place the palmar aspect of your left forearm against the patient's sacrum and posterior superior iliac spine. Rotate the patient's pelvis and lumbar spine towards you until motion is palpated at the T12–L1 segment. Rotate the patient's upper body away from you until a sense of tension is palpated at the T12–L1 segment. Roll the patient about 10–15° towards you

- **Adjustments to achieve appropriate pre-thrust tension**

- **Immediately pre-thrust:** Relax and adjust your balance

- **Delivering the thrust:** The direction of thrust is down towards the couch accompanied by exaggeration of pelvic rotation towards the operator (Fig. 10.16). Your right arm against the patient's axillary region does not apply a thrust but acts as a stabilizer only

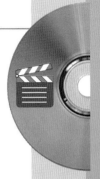

Lumbar spine L1–5
Neutral positioning

Patient sidelying
Rotation gliding thrust

Assume somatic dysfunction (S-T-A-R-T) is identified and you wish to use a rotation gliding thrust to produce cavitation at L3–4 on the right (Figs 10.17, 10.18).

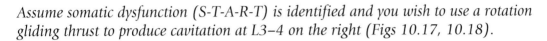

Figure 10.17

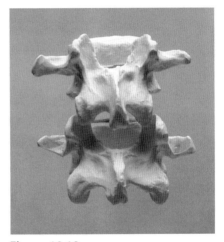

Figure 10.18

KEY

✳ Stabilization

● Applicator

→ Plane of thrust (operator)

⇨ Direction of body movement (patient)

Note: The dimensions for the arrows are not a pictorial representation of the amplitude or force of the thrust.

1. **Patient positioning**

Lying on the left side with a pillow to support the head and neck.

Lower body. Straighten the patient's lower leg and ensure that the leg and spine are in a straight line, in a neutral position. Flex the patient's upper hip and knee slightly and place the upper leg just anterior to the lower leg. The lower leg and spine should form as near a straight line as possible, with no flexion at the lower hip or knee.

Upper body. Gently extend the patient's upper shoulder and place the patient's right forearm on the lower ribs. Using your left hand to palpate the L3–4 interspinous space, introduce right rotation of the patient's upper body down to the L3–4 segment. This is

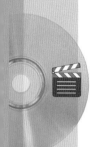

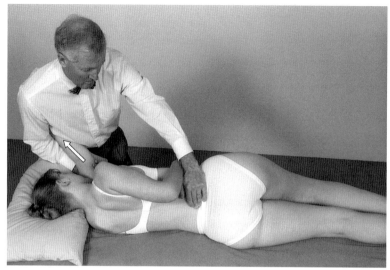

Figure 10.19

achieved by gently holding the patient's left elbow with your right hand and pulling it towards you, but also in a cephalad direction towards the head end of the couch (Fig. 10.19). Be careful not to introduce any flexion to the spine during this movement. Right rotation is continued until your palpating hand at the L3–4 segment begins to sense motion. Take up the axillary hold. This arm controls the upper body rotation.

2. **Operator stance**

Stand close to the couch with your feet spread and one leg behind the other (Fig. 10.20). Maintain an upright posture, facing slightly in the direction of the patient's upper body. Keep your left arm as close to your body as possible.

3. **Positioning for thrust**

Apply your left forearm to the region between gluteus medius and maximus. Your left forearm now controls lower body rotation. Your right forearm should be resting against the patient's upper pectoral and rib cage region and will control upper body rotation. First, rotate the patient's pelvis and lumbar spine towards you until motion is palpated at the L3–4 segment. Rotate the patient's upper body away from you using your right arm until a sense of tension is palpated at the L3–4

segment. Be careful to avoid undue pressure in the axilla. Finally, roll the patient about 10–15° towards you while maintaining the build-up of leverages at the L3–4 segment.

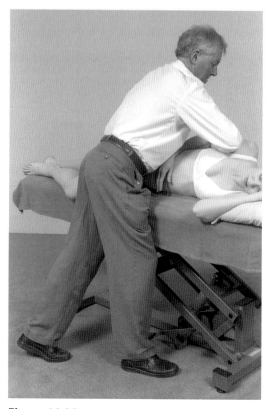

Figure 10.20

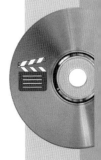

4. **Adjustments to achieve appropriate pre-thrust tension**

Ensure your patient remains relaxed. Maintaining all holds, make any necessary changes in flexion, extension, sidebending or rotation until you can sense a state of appropriate tension and leverage at the L3–4 segment. The patient should not be aware of any pain or discomfort. Make these final adjustments by slight movements of the shoulders, trunk, ankles, knees and hips.

5. **Immediately pre-thrust**

Relax and adjust your balance as necessary. Keep your head up; looking down impedes the thrust. An effective HVLA thrust technique is best achieved if both the operator and patient are relaxed and not holding themselves rigid.

This is a common impediment to achieving effective cavitation.

6. **Delivering the thrust**

Your right arm against the patient's pectoral region does not apply a thrust but acts as a stabilizer only. Keep the thrusting (left) arm as close to your body as possible. Apply a HVLA thrust with your left forearm against the patient's buttock. The direction of force is down towards the couch accompanied by slight exaggeration of pelvic rotation towards the operator (Fig. 10.21).

The thrust, although very rapid, must never be excessively forcible. The aim should be to use the absolute minimum force necessary to achieve joint cavitation. A common fault arises from the use of excessive amplitude with insufficient velocity of thrust.

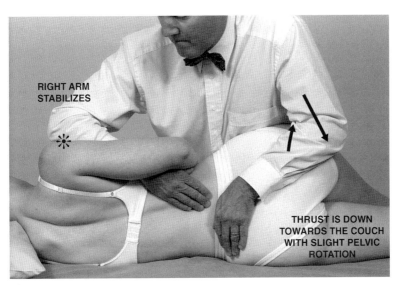

RIGHT ARM STABILIZES

THRUST IS DOWN TOWARDS THE COUCH WITH SLIGHT PELVIC ROTATION

Figure 10.21

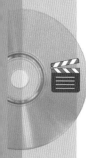

SUMMARY

Lumbar spine L1–5 Neutral positioning

Patient sidelying

Rotation gliding thrust

- **Patient positioning:** Left sidelying:

  Lower body. Left leg and spine in a straight line. Right hip and knee flexed slightly and placed just anterior to the lower leg

  Upper body. Introduce right rotation of the patient's upper body until your palpating hand at L3–4 begins to sense motion. Do not introduce any flexion to the spine during this movement (Fig. 10.19). Take up the axillary hold

- **Operator stance:** Stand close to the couch, feet spread and one leg behind the other. Maintain an upright posture, facing slightly in the direction of the patient's upper body (Fig. 10.20)

- **Positioning for thrust:** Place your left forearm in the region between gluteus medius and maximus. Rotate the patient's pelvis and lumbar spine towards you until motion is palpated at the L3–4 segment. Rotate the patient's upper body away from you until a sense of tension is palpated at the L3–4 segment. Roll the patient about 10–15° towards you

- **Adjustments to achieve appropriate pre-thrust tension**

- **Immediately pre-thrust:** Relax and adjust your balance

- **Delivering the thrust:** The direction of thrust is down towards the couch accompanied by exaggeration of pelvic rotation towards the operator (Fig. 10.21). Your right arm against the patient's axillary region does not apply a thrust but acts as a stabilizer only

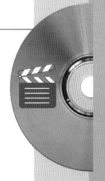

Lumbar spine L1–5
Flexion positioning

Patient sidelying
Rotation gliding thrust

Assume somatic dysfunction (S-T-A-R-T) is identified and you wish to use a rotation gliding thrust to produce cavitation at L3–4 on the right (Figs 10.22, 10.23).

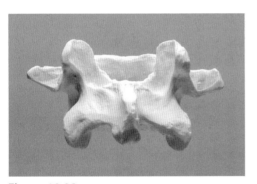

Figure 10.22

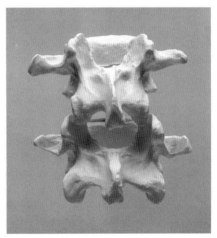

Figure 10.23

KEY

✳ Stabilization

● Applicator

➜ Plane of thrust (operator)

⇨ Direction of body movement (patient)

Note: The dimensions for the arrows are not a pictorial representation of the amplitude or force of the thrust.

1. Patient positioning

Lying on the left side with a pillow to support the head and neck. A small pillow, or rolled towel, should be placed under the patient's waist to introduce left sidebending in the lumbar spine. Experienced practitioners may choose to achieve the left sidebending without the use of a small pillow or rolled towel.

Lower body. Straighten the patient's lower (left) leg at the knee joint while keeping the left hip flexed. Flex the patient's upper hip and knee. Rest the upper flexed knee upon the edge of the couch, anterior to the left thigh, and place the patient's right foot behind the left calf. This position provides stability to the lower body.

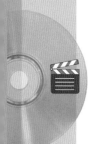

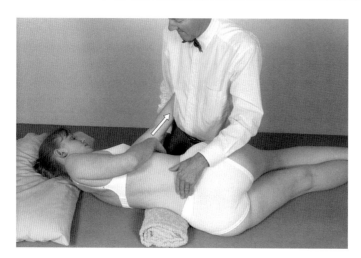

Figure 10.24

Upper body. Gently extend the patient's upper shoulder and place the patient's right forearm on the lower ribs. Using your left hand to palpate the L3–4 interspinous space, introduce right rotation of the patient's upper body down to the L3–4 segment. Rotation with flexion positioning is achieved by gently holding the patient's left elbow with your right hand and pulling it towards you, but also in a caudad direction towards the foot end of the couch (Fig. 10.24). Right rotation is continued until your palpating hand at the L3–4 segment begins to sense motion. Take up the axillary hold. This arm controls the upper body rotation.

2. **Operator stance**

Stand close to the couch with your feet spread and one leg behind the other (Fig. 10.25). Maintain an upright posture, facing slightly in the direction of the patient's upper body. Keep your left arm as close to your body as possible.

3. **Positioning for thrust**

Apply your left forearm to the region between gluteus medius and maximus. Your left forearm now controls lower body rotation. Your right forearm should be resting against the patient's upper pectoral and rib cage region and will control upper body rotation. First, rotate the patient's pelvis and lumbar spine towards you until motion is palpated at the L3–4 segment. Rotate the patient's upper

body away from you using your right arm until a sense of tension is palpated at the L3–4 segment. Be careful to avoid undue pressure in the axilla. Finally, roll the patient about 10–15° towards you while maintaining the build-up of leverages at the L3–4 segment.

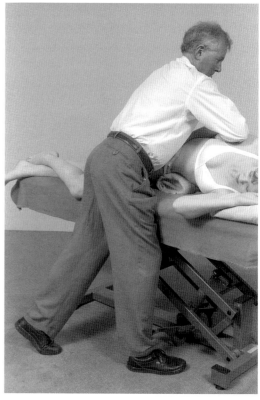

Figure 10.25

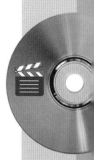

4. Adjustments to achieve appropriate pre-thrust tension

Ensure your patient remains relaxed. Maintaining all holds, make any necessary changes in flexion, extension, sidebending or rotation until you can sense a state of appropriate tension and leverage at the L3–4 segment. The patient should not be aware of any pain or discomfort. Make these final adjustments by slight movements of the shoulders, trunk, ankles, knees and hips.

5. Immediately pre-thrust

Relax and adjust your balance as necessary. Keep your head up; looking down impedes the thrust. An effective HVLA thrust technique is best achieved if both the operator and patient are relaxed and not holding themselves rigid.

This is a common impediment to achieving effective cavitation.

6. Delivering the thrust

Your right arm against the patient's pectoral region does not apply a thrust but acts as a stabilizer only. Keep the thrusting (left) arm as close to your body as possible. Apply a HVLA thrust with your left forearm against the patient's buttock. The direction of force is down towards the couch accompanied by a slight exaggeration of pelvic rotation towards the operator (Fig. 10.26).

The thrust, although very rapid, must never be excessively forcible. The aim should be to use the absolute minimum force necessary to achieve joint cavitation. A common fault arises from the use of excessive amplitude with insufficient velocity of thrust.

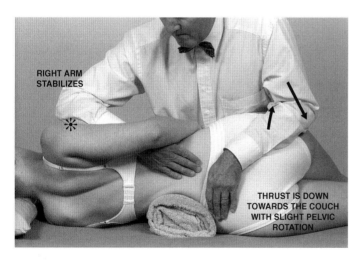

RIGHT ARM
STABILIZES

THRUST IS DOWN
TOWARDS THE COUCH
WITH SLIGHT PELVIC
ROTATION

Figure 10.26

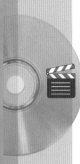

SUMMARY

Lumbar spine L1–5 Flexion positioning

Patient sidelying

Rotation gliding thrust

- **Patient positioning:** Left sidelying with a small pillow or rolled towel placed under the patient's waist to introduce left sidebending in the lumbar spine:

  Lower body. Left hip flexed with knee extended. Right hip and knee flexed with the patient's right foot behind the left calf

  Upper body. Introduce right rotation of the patient's upper body until your palpating hand at L3–4 begins to sense motion. Introduce flexion to the spine during this movement (Fig. 10.24). Take up the axillary hold

- **Operator stance:** Stand close to the couch, feet spread and one leg behind the other. Maintain an upright posture, facing slightly in the direction of the patient's upper body (Fig. 10.25)

- **Positioning for thrust:** Place your left forearm in the region between gluteus medius and maximus. Rotate the patient's pelvis and lumbar spine towards you until motion is palpated at the L3–4 segment. Rotate the patient's upper body away from you until a sense of tension is palpated at the L3–4 segment. Roll the patient about 10–15° towards you

- **Adjustments to achieve appropriate pre-thrust tension**

- **Immediately pre-thrust:** Relax and adjust your balance

- **Delivering the thrust:** The direction of thrust is down towards the couch accompanied by exaggeration of pelvic rotation towards the operator (Fig. 10.26). Your right arm against the patient's axillary region does not apply a thrust but acts as a stabilizer only

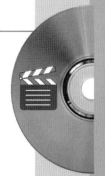

Lumbar spine L1–5
Neutral positioning

Patient sitting
Rotation gliding thrust

Assume somatic dysfunction (S-T-A-R-T) is identified and you wish to use a rotation gliding thrust to produce cavitation at L3–4 on the left (Figs 10.27, 10.28).

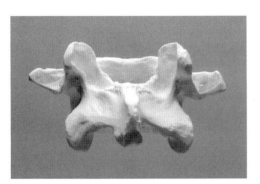

Figure 10.27

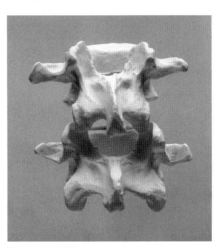

Figure 10.28

KEY

 Stabilization

● Applicator

→ Plane of thrust (operator)

⇨ Direction of body movement (patient)

Note: The dimensions for the arrows are not a pictorial representation of the amplitude or force of the thrust.

1. **Patient positioning**

Sitting on the treatment couch with the arms folded. The patient should be encouraged to maintain an erect posture.

2. **Operator stance**

Stand behind and slightly to the right of the patient with your feet spread. Pass your right arm across the front of the patient's chest to lightly grip the patient's left thorax (Fig. 10.29).

3. **Positioning for thrust**

Place your left hypothenar eminence to the right side of the spinous process of L3 and introduce right sidebending to the patient's

237

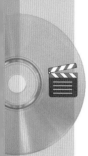

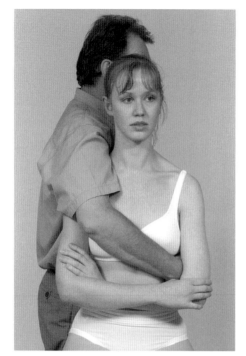

Figure 10.29

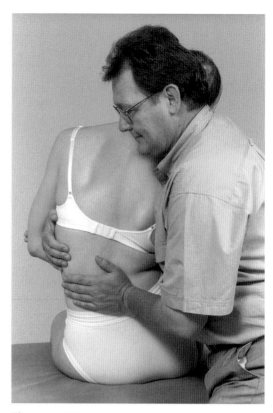

Figure 10.30

thoracic and upper lumbar spine (Fig. 10.30). The thoracic and upper lumbar spine is now rotated to the right to lock the spine down to but not including L3–4. The operator maintains as erect a posture as possible. Keep your left hypothenar eminence firmly applied to the spinous process of L3 with your left arm held close to your body.

4. Adjustments to achieve appropriate pre-thrust tension

Ensure your patient remains relaxed. Maintaining all holds, make any necessary changes in flexion, extension, sidebending or rotation until you can sense a state of appropriate tension and leverage at the

L3–4 segment. The patient should not be aware of any pain or discomfort. Make these final adjustments by slight movements of the shoulders, trunk, ankles, knees and hips.

5. Immediately pre-thrust

Relax and adjust your balance as necessary. An effective HVLA thrust technique is best achieved if both the operator and patient are relaxed and not holding themselves rigid. This is a common impediment to achieving effective cavitation.

6. Delivering the thrust

A degree of momentum is necessary to achieve a successful cavitation. It is desirable for the momentum component of the thrust to be restricted to one plane of motion and this should be rotation. Rock the patient into and out of rotation while maintaining the sidebending and flexion / extension positioning. When close to full rotation, you will sense a state of appropriate tension and leverage at the L3–4 segment, at which point you apply a HVLA thrust against the spinous process of L3. The thrust is directed to the spinous process of L3 and accompanied by a slight exaggeration of right rotation (Fig. 10.31).

The thrust, although very rapid, must never be excessively forcible. The aim should be to use the absolute minimum force necessary to achieve joint cavitation. A common fault arises from the use of excessive amplitude with insufficient velocity of thrust.

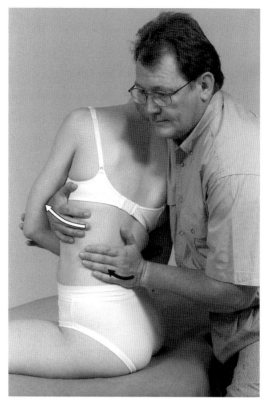
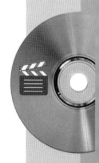

Figure 10.31

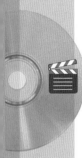

SUMMARY

Lumbar spine L1–5 Neutral positioning

Patient sitting

Rotation gliding thrust

- **Patient positioning:** Sitting erect
- **Operator stance:** Behind and slightly to the right of the patient with your right arm across the front of the patient's chest (Fig. 10.29)
- **Positioning for thrust:** Place your left hypothenar eminence to the right side of the spinous process of L3 and introduce right sidebending to the patient's thoracic and upper lumbar spine (Fig. 10.30). The thoracic and upper lumbar spine is now rotated to the right to lock the spine down to but not including L3–4
- **Adjustments to achieve appropriate pre-thrust tension**
- **Immediately pre-thrust:** Relax and adjust your balance
- **Delivering the thrust:** The thrust is directed to the spinous process of L3 and accompanied by exaggeration of right rotation (Fig. 10.31). A degree of momentum is necessary to achieve a successful cavitation. The momentum component of the thrust should be in the direction of rotation.

Lumbosacral joint (L5–S1)
Neutral positioning

Patient sidelying

Thrust direction is dependent upon apophysial joint plane[†]

Assume somatic dysfunction (S-T-A-R-T) is identified and you wish to use a gliding thrust to produce cavitation at L5–S1 on the right (Figs 10.32, 10.33).

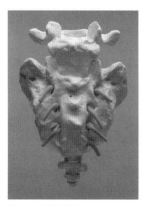

Figure 10.32

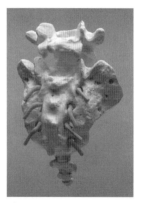

Figure 10.33

KEY

❋ Stabilization

● Applicator

→ Plane of thrust (operator)

⇨ Direction of body movement (patient)

Note: The dimensions for the arrows are not a pictorial representation of the amplitude or force of the thrust.

1. Patient positioning

Lying on the left side with a pillow to support the head and neck.

Lower body. Straighten the patient's lower (left) leg at the knee joint while placing the

[†] The condition where joints are asymmetrically orientated is referred to as articular tropism. The lumbosacral zygapophysial joints would normally be orientated at approximately 45° with respect to the sagittal plane. There is considerable individual variation and you will encounter patients with lumbosacral apophysial joint planes that range between sagittal and coronal orientation. The variation in apophysial joint plane means that considerable palpatory skill is required to localize forces accurately at the lumbosacral joint and to determine the most suitable direction of thrust.

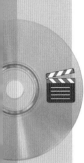

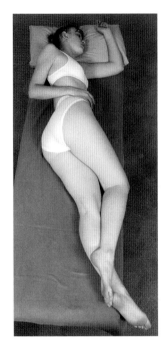

Figure 10.34

left hip in approximately 20° of flexion. Flex the patient's upper knee and place the patient's right foot behind the left lower leg (Fig. 10.34). This position provides stability to the lower body.

Upper body. Gently extend the patient's upper shoulder and place the patient's right forearm on the lower ribs. Using your left hand to palpate the L5–S1 interspinous space, introduce right rotation of the patient's upper body down to the L5–S1 segment. This is achieved by gently holding the patient's left elbow with your right hand and pulling it towards you, but also in a cephalad direction towards the head end of the couch. Be careful not to introduce any flexion to the spine during this movement. Right rotation is continued until your palpating hand at the L5–S1 segment begins to sense motion. Take up the axillary hold. This arm controls the upper body rotation.

2. **Operator stance**

Stand close to the couch with your feet spread and one leg behind the other. Maintain an

upright posture, facing slightly in the direction of the patient's upper body. Keep your left arm as close to your body as possible.

3. **Positioning for thrust**

Apply your left forearm to the region between gluteus medius and maximus. Your left forearm now controls lower body rotation. Your right forearm rests on the patient's right axillary area. This will control upper body rotation. First, apply pressure to the patient's pelvis until motion is palpated at the L5–S1 segment. Rotate the patient's upper body away from you using your right arm until a sense of tension is palpated at the L5–S1 segment. Finally, roll the patient about 10–15° towards you while maintaining the build-up of leverages at the L5–S1segment.

4. **Adjustments to achieve appropriate pre-thrust tension**

Ensure your patient remains relaxed. Maintaining all holds, make any necessary changes in flexion, extension, sidebending or rotation until you can sense a state of appropriate tension and leverage at the L5–S1 segment. The patient should not be aware of any pain or discomfort. Make these final adjustments by slight movements of the shoulders, trunk, ankles, knees and hips.

5. **Immediately pre-thrust**

Relax and adjust your balance as necessary. Keep your head up; looking down impedes the thrust. An effective HVLA thrust technique is best achieved if both the operator and patient are relaxed and not holding themselves rigid. This is a common impediment to achieving effective cavitation.

6. **Delivering the thrust**

Your right arm against the patient's axillary region does not apply a thrust but acts as a stabilizer only (Fig. 10.35). Keep the thrusting (left) arm as close to your body as possible. Apply a HVLA thrust with your left forearm against the patient's buttock. The direction of

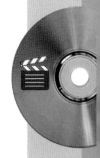

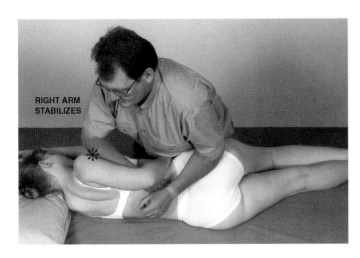

RIGHT ARM
STABILIZES

Figure 10.35

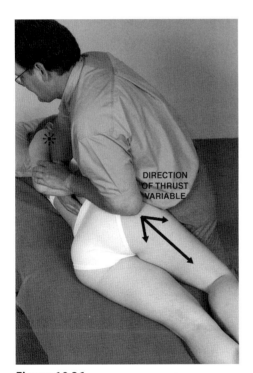

DIRECTION
OF THRUST
VARIABLE

Figure 10.36

thrust is variable depending on the apophysial joint plane. Commonly the direction of thrust approximates to a line along the long axis of the patient's right femur (Fig. 10.36).

The thrust, although very rapid, must never be excessively forcible. The aim should be to use the absolute minimum force necessary to achieve joint cavitation. A common fault arises from the use of excessive amplitude with insufficient velocity of thrust.

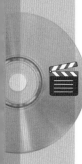

SUMMARY

Lumbosacral Joint (L5–S1) Neutral positioning

Patient sidelying

Thrust direction is dependent upon apophysial joint plane

- **Patient positioning:** Left sidelying:

  Lower body. Left hip in approximately 20° of flexion with knee extended. Right hip and knee flexed (Fig. 10.34)

  Upper body. Introduce right rotation of the patient's upper body until your palpating hand at the L5–S1 segment begins to sense motion. Do not introduce any flexion to the spine during this movement. Take up the axillary hold

- **Operator stance:** Stand close to the couch, feet spread and one leg behind the other. Maintain an upright posture, facing slightly in the direction of the patient's upper body

- **Positioning for thrust:** Place your left forearm in the region between gluteus medius and maximus. Apply pressure to the patient's pelvis until motion is palpated at the L5–S1 segment. Rotate the patient's upper body away from you until a sense of tension is palpated at the L5–S1 segment. Roll the patient about 10–15° towards you

- **Adjustments to achieve appropriate pre-thrust tension**

- **Immediately pre-thrust:** Relax and adjust your balance

- **Delivering the thrust:** Your right arm against the patient's axillary region does not apply a thrust but acts as a stabilizer only (Fig. 10.35). The direction of thrust is variable depending on the apophysial joint plane. Commonly the thrust is along the long axis of the patient's right femur (Fig. 10.36)

10.7

Lumbosacral joint (L5–S1)
Flexion positioning

Patient sidelying
Thrust direction is dependent upon apophysial joint plane[†]

Assume somatic dysfunction (S-T-A-R-T) is identified and you wish to use a gliding thrust to produce cavitation at L5–S1 on the right (Figs 10.37, 10.38).

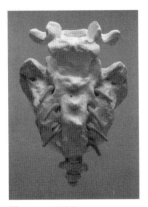

Figure 10.37

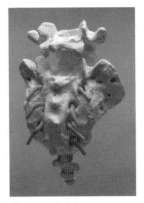

Figure 10.38

KEY

✷ Stabilization

● Applicator

➜ Plane of thrust (operator)

⇨ Direction of body movement (patient)

Note: The dimensions for the arrows are not a pictorial representation of the amplitude or force of the thrust.

1. Patient positioning

Lying on the left side with a pillow to support the head and neck.

Lower body. Straighten the patient's lower (left) leg at the knee joint while placing the

[†] The condition where joints are asymmetrically orientated is referred to as articular tropism. The lumbosacral zygapophysial joints would normally be orientated at approximately 45° with respect to the sagittal plane. There is considerable individual variation and you will encounter patients with lumbosacral apophysial joint planes that range between sagittal and coronal orientation. The variation in apophysial joint plane means that considerable palpatory skill is required to localize forces accurately at the lumbosacral joint and to determine the most suitable direction of thrust.

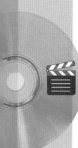

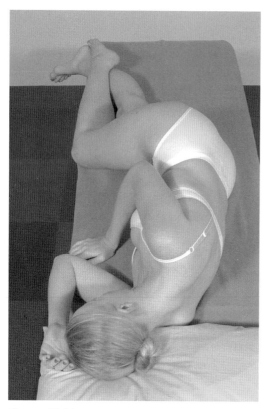

Figure 10.39

left hip in approximately 20° of flexion. Flex the patient's upper knee and place the patient's right foot behind the left lower leg (Fig. 10.39). This position provides stability to the lower body.

Upper body. Gently extend the patient's upper shoulder and place the patient's right forearm on the lower ribs. Using your left hand to palpate the L5–S1 interspinous space, introduce right rotation of the patient's upper body down to the L5–S1 segment. Rotation with flexion positioning is achieved by gently holding the patient's left elbow with your right hand and pulling it towards you, but also in a caudad direction towards the foot end of the couch. Right rotation is continued until your palpating hand at the L5–S1 segment begins to sense motion. Take up the axillary hold. This arm controls the upper body rotation.

2. **Operator stance**

Stand close to the couch with your feet spread and one leg behind the other. Maintain an upright posture, facing slightly in the direction of the patient's upper body. Keep your left arm as close to your body as possible.

3. **Positioning for thrust**

Apply your left forearm to the region between gluteus medius and maximus. Your left forearm now controls lower body rotation. Your right forearm rests on the patient's right axillary area. This will control upper body rotation. First, apply pressure to the patient's pelvis until motion is palpated at the L5–S1 segment. Introduce left sidebending to lumbar spine by applying pressure with the left forearm to the patient's pelvis in a caudad direction (Fig. 10.40). Now rotate the patient's upper body away from you using your right arm until a sense of tension is palpated at the L5–S1 segment. Finally, roll the patient about 10–15° towards you while maintaining the build-up of leverages at the L5–S1 segment.

4. **Adjustments to achieve appropriate pre-thrust tension**

Ensure your patient remains relaxed. Maintaining all holds, make any necessary changes in flexion, extension, sidebending or rotation until you can sense a state of appropriate tension and leverage at the L5–S1 segment. The patient should not be aware of any pain or discomfort. Make these final adjustments by slight movements of the shoulders, trunk, ankles, knees and hips.

5. **Immediately pre-thrust**

Relax and adjust your balance as necessary. Keep your head up; looking down impedes the thrust. An effective HVLA thrust technique is best achieved if both the operator and patient are relaxed and not holding themselves rigid. This is a common impediment to achieving effective cavitation.

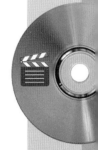

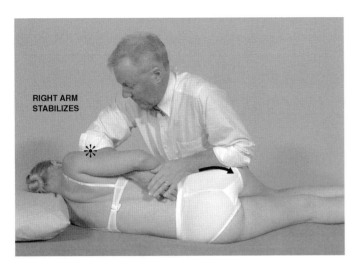

RIGHT ARM
STABILIZES

Figure 10.40

6. Delivering the thrust

Your right arm against the patient's axillary region does not apply a thrust but acts as a stabilizer only. Keep the thrusting (left) arm as close to your body as possible and maintain the left lumbar sidebending leverage. Apply a HVLA thrust with your left forearm against the patient's buttock. The direction of thrust is variable depending on the apophysial joint plane. Commonly the direction of thrust approximates to a line along the long axis of the patient's right femur (Fig. 10.41).

The thrust, although very rapid, must never be excessively forcible. The aim should be to use the absolute minimum of force necessary to achieve joint cavitation. A common fault arises from the use of excessive amplitude with insufficient velocity of thrust.

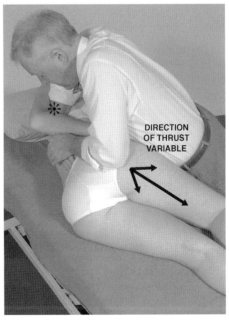

DIRECTION
OF THRUST
VARIABLE

Figure 10.41

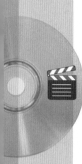

SUMMARY

Lumbosacral joint (L5–S1) Flexion positioning

Patient sidelying

Thrust direction is dependent upon apophysial joint plane

- **Patient positioning:** Left sidelying:

  Lower body. Left hip in approximately 20° of flexion with knee extended. Right hip and knee flexed (Fig. 10.39)

  Upper body. Introduce right rotation of the patient's upper body until your palpating hand at the L5–S1 segment begins to sense motion. Introduce flexion to the spine during this movement. Take up the axillary hold

- **Operator stance:** Stand close to the couch, feet spread and one leg behind the other. Maintain an upright posture, facing slightly in the direction of the patient's upper body

- **Positioning for thrust:** Place your left forearm in the region between gluteus medius and maximus. Apply pressure to the patient's pelvis until motion is palpated at the L5–S1 segment. Sidebend the lumbar spine to the left (Fig. 10.40) and then rotate the patient's upper body away from you until a sense of tension is palpated at the L5–S1 segment. Roll the patient about 10–15° towards you

- **Adjustments to achieve appropriate pre-thrust tension**

- **Immediately pre-thrust:** Relax and adjust your balance

- **Delivering the thrust:** Your right arm against the patient's axillary region does not apply a thrust but acts as a stabilizer only. It is critical to maintain left lumbar sidebending when delivering the thrust. The direction of thrust is variable depending on the apophysial joint plane. Commonly the thrust is along the long axis of the patient's right femur (Fig. 10.41)

11

Pelvis

INTRODUCTION

The sacroiliac joint as a source of pain and dysfunction is a subject of controversy.[1-6] Many authors implicate the sacroiliac joint as a cause of low back pain,[6-19] but there is disagreement as to the exact prevalence of sacroiliac joint pain within the low back pain population. It is estimated that 5–15% of chronic low back pain may involve the sacroiliac joint.[14,16,20] Although many practitioners believe the sacroiliac joint is a source of pain and dysfunction and treat perceived sacroiliac lesions, there is no general agreement concerning the different diagnostic tests and their validity in determining somatic dysfunction of the pelvis (Fig. 11.1).[16,21-33] Assessment of the sacroiliac joint in the male population may be confounded by joint fusion, which is present in 5.8% of males up to the age of 39 increasing to 46.7% of males over 80 years of age.[34]

A large number of diagnostic tests exist to evaluate the sacroiliac joint. Motion tests and static palpation of bony landmarks have generally shown poor inter-observer reliability. Pain provocation tests have shown better reliability,[35] with clusters of pain provocation tests showing even greater reliability.[35-38] Arab et al[39] suggest that composites of motion palpation and provocation tests may be useful in clinical practice. Laslett[40] suggests that the combination of non-centralization of pain on repeated trunk movements with three or more sacroiliac joint provocation tests that reproduce the patient's familiar pain might help to differentiate sacroiliac joint pain from other painful conditions.

Various models of sacroiliac motion have been proposed and there have been a number of studies relating to mobility in the sacroiliac joint,[41-48] but the precise nature of normal motion remains unclear.[1,4,17,49,50] There is

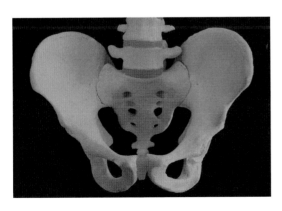

Figure 11.1 The pelvic girdle.

significant variation in sacroiliac joint movement both between individuals and within individuals when mobility of one sacroiliac joint is compared with the other side.[43] Mobility alters with age and can increase during pregnancy.

At our present state of knowledge, what model should guide our clinical decision making to incorporate high-velocity low-amplitude (HVLA) thrust techniques within a treatment regimen for somatic dysfunction of the pelvis? There are a number of different biomechanical models used to determine the nature of any pelvic dysfunction.[51–55] These vary from very complex to less complex with no research evidence as to their clinical utility. Greenman[54] describes a number of possible pelvic girdle dysfunctions, which are listed in Box 11.1.

A number of manual medicine texts[56–61] refer to the use of HVLA thrust techniques to the joints of the pelvis, but there is little

evidence that cavitation is uniformly associated with these procedures. When an audible release does occur, its site of origin remains open to speculation. Studies undertaken to measure the effects of manipulation upon the sacroiliac joints provide contradictory findings. Roentgen stereophotogrammetric analysis was unable to detect altered position of the sacroiliac joint post manipulation despite normalization of different types of clinical tests.[62] However, an alteration in pelvic tilt was identified post manipulation in one study of patients with low back pain[63] and a further study demonstrated an immediate improvement in iliac crest symmetry immediately after manipulation.[64] A review of the literature did not reveal any randomized controlled trials investigating the use of HVLA thrust techniques for pelvic girdle pain.

Many practitioners believe that HVLA thrust techniques applied to the sacroiliac joint can be associated with good clinical outcomes. As a result, many clinicians continue to use HVLA thrust techniques to treat somatic dysfunction of the joints of the pelvis.

Somatic dysfunction is identified by the S-T-A-R-T of diagnosis:

- S relates to symptom reproduction
- T relates to tissue tenderness
- A relates to asymmetry
- R relates to range of motion
- T relates to tissue texture changes

Chapter 11 describes in detail four HVLA thrust techniques for the sacroiliac joint and one for the sacrococcygeal joint. All the techniques are described using a variable-height manipulation couch.

After making a diagnosis of somatic dysfunction and prior to proceeding with a thrust, it is recommended the following checklist be used for each of the techniques described in this chapter:

- Have I excluded all contraindications?
- Have I explained to the patient what I am going to do?

Box 11.1 Pelvic girdle dysfunctions

Pubis
1. Superior
2. Inferior

Sacroiliac
1. Bilaterally nutated anteriorly
2. Bilaterally nutated posteriorly
3. Unilaterally nutated anteriorly (sacrum flexed)
4. Unilaterally nutated posteriorly (sacrum extended)
5. Torsioned anteriorly (left on left or right on right)
6. Torsioned posteriorly (left on right or right on left)

Iliosacral
1. Rotated anteriorly
2. Rotated posteriorly
3. Superior (cephalic) shear
4. Inferior (caudad) shear
5. Rotated medially (inflare)
6. Rotated laterally (outflare)

Reproduced with permission from Greenman.[54]

- Do I have informed consent?
- Is the patient well positioned and comfortable?
- Am I in a comfortable and balanced position?
- Do I need to modify any pre-thrust physical or biomechanical factors?
- Have I achieved appropriate pre-thrust tissue tension?
- Am I relaxed and confident to proceed?
- Is the patient relaxed and willing for me to proceed?

References

1 Alderink GJ. The sacroiliac joint: review of anatomy, mechanics, and function. J Orthop Sports Phys Ther 1991;13:71–84.

2 Bernard TN, Cassidy JD. The sacroiliac joint syndrome – pathophysiology, diagnosis and management. In: Frymoyer J W ed. The Adult Spine: Principles and Practice. New York, NY: Raven Press; 1991:2107–2130.

3 Walker JM. The sacroiliac joint: a critical review. Phys Ther 1992;72:903–916.

4 Dreyfuss P, Cole AJ, Pauza K. Sacroiliac joint injection techniques. Phys Med Rehabil Clin North Am 1995;6(4):785–813.

5 Cibulka M. Understanding sacroiliac joint movement as a guide to the management of a patient with unilateral low back pain. Man Ther 2002;7(4):215–221.

6 Brolinson P, Kozar A, Cibor G. Sacroiliac joint dysfunction in athletes. Curr Sports Med Rep 2003;2(1):47–56.

7 Grieve G. The sacroiliac joint. Physiotherapy 1976;62:384–400.

8 Weismantel A. Evaluation and treatment of sacroiliac joint problems. J Am Phys Ther Assoc 1978;3(1):1–9.

9 Mitchell F. Vol 1. The Muscle Energy Manual. East Lansing, MI: MET Press; 1995.

10 DonTigny RL. Function and pathomechanics of the sacroiliac joint. Phys Ther 1985;65:35–43.

11 Bernard TN, Kirkaldy-Willis WH. Recognizing specific characteristics of nonspecific low back pain. Clin Orthop 1987;217:266–280.

12 Bourdillon JF, Day EA, Boohout MR. Spinal Manipulation, 5th edn. Avon: Bath Press; 1995.

13 Shaw JL. The role of the sacroiliac joint as a cause of low back pain and dysfunction. First Interdisciplinary World Congress on Low Back Pain and its Relation to the Sacroiliac Joint. Rotterdam: ECO; 1992.

14 Schwarzer AC, Aprill CN, Bogduk N. The sacroiliac joint in chronic low back pain. Spine 1995;20:31–37.

15 Herzog W. Clinical Biomechanics of Spinal Manipulation. New York: Churchill Livingstone; 2000.

16 Maigne JY, Aivaliklis A, Pfefer F. Results of sacroiliac joint double block and value of sacroiliac pain provocation tests in 54 patients with low back pain. Spine 1996;21(16): 1889–1892.

17 Foley B, Buschbacher R. Sacroiliac joint pain: Anatomy, biomechanics, diagnosis, and treatment. Am J Phys Med Rehabil 2006;85(12): 997–1006.

18 Forst S, Wheeler M, Fortin J, et al. The sacroiliac joint: anatomy, physiology and clinical significance. Pain Physician 2006; 9(1):61–67.

19 Hansen H, McKenzie-Brown A, Cohen S, et al. Sacroiliac joint interventions: a systematic review. Pain Physician 2007;10(1):165–184.

20 Hansen H, Helm S. Sacroiliac joint pain and dysfunction. Pain Physician 2003;6(2): 179–189.

21 Speed C. ABC of Rheumatology. Low back pain. BMJ 2004;328:1119–1121.

22 Carmichael JP. Inter and intra-examiner reliability of palpation for sacroiliac joint dysfunction. J Manipulative Physiol Ther 1987;10:164–171.

23 Dreyfuss P, Dreyer S, Griffin J, et al. Positive sacroiliac screening tests in asymptomatic adults. Spine 1994;19:1138–1143.

24 Dreyfuss P, Michaelsen M, Pauza K, et al. The value of medical history and physical examination in diagnosing sacroiliac joint pain. Spine 1996;21:2594–2602.

25 Herzog W, Read L, Conway P, et al. Reliability of motion palpation procedures to detect sacro-iliac joint fixations. J Manipulative Physiol Ther 1988;11:151–157.

26 Laslett M, Williams M. The reliability of selected pain provocation tests for sacroiliac joint pathology. Spine 1994;19:1243–1249.

27 Van Deursen LLJM, Patijn J, Ockhuysen AL, et al. The value of some clinical tests of the sacro-iliac joint. Man Med 1990;5:96–99.

28 Riddle D, Freburger J. Evaluation of the presence of sacroiliac joint region dysfunction using a combination of tests: A multicenter intertester reliability study. Phys Ther 2002;82(8):772–781.

29 Young S, Aprill C, Laslett M. Correlation of clinical examination characteristics with three sources of chronic low back pain. Spine 2003; 3(6):460–465.

30 Meijne W, van Neerbos K, Aufdemkampe G, et al. Intraexaminer and interexaminer reliability of the Gillet test. J Manipulative Physiol Ther 1999;22(1):4–9.

31 Sturesson B, Uden A, Vleeming A. A radiostereometric analysis of the movements of the sacroiliac joints during the standing hip flexion test. Spine 2000;25(3):364–368.

32 Vincent-Smith B, Gibbons P. Inter-examiner and intra-examiner reliability of palpatory findings for the standing flexion test. Man Ther 1999;4 (2):87–93.

33 O'Haire C, Gibbons P. Inter-examiner and intra-examiner agreement for assessing sacro-iliac anatomical landmarks using palpation and observation: A pilot study. Man Ther 2000;5(1): 13–20.

34 Dar G, Khamis S, Peleg S, et al. Sacroiliac joint fusion and the implications for manual therapy diagnosis and treatment. Man Ther 2008;13(2): 155–158.

35 Laslett M, Aprill C, McDonald B, et al. Diagnosis of sacroiliac joint pain: validity of individual provocation tests and composites of tests. Man Ther 2005;10(3):207–218.

36 Kokmeyer D, van der Wurff P, et al. The reliability of multitest regimens with sacroiliac pain provocation tests. J Manipulative Physiol Ther 2002;25(1):42–48.

37 van der Wurff P, Buijs E, Groen G. A multitest regimen of pain provocation tests as an aid to reduce unnecessary minimally invasive sacroiliac joint procedures. Arch Phys Med Rehabil 2006;87(1):10–14.

38 Robinson H, Brox J, Robinson R, et al. The reliability of selected motion and pain provocation tests for the sacroiliac joint. Man Ther 2007;12(1):72–79.

39 Arab A, Abdollahi I, Joghataei T, et al. Inter- and intra-examiner reliability of single and composites of selected motion palpation and pain provocation tests for sacroiliac joint. Man Ther 2009;14(2):213–221.

40 Laslett M. Pain provocation tests for diagnosis of sacroiliac joint pain. Aust J Physiother 2006; 52(3):229.

41 Colachis SC, Worden RE, Brechtol CO, et al. Movement of the sacroiliac joint in the adult male: a preliminary report. Arch Phys Med Rehabil 1963;44:490–498.

42 Egund N, Olsson TH, Schmid H, et al. Movements in the sacroiliac joints demonstrated with Roentgen stereophotogrammetry. Acta Radiol Diagn 1978;19:833–846.

43 Sturesson B, Selvik G, Uden A. Movements of the sacroiliac joints. A Roentgen stereophotogrammetric analysis. Spine 1989;14:162–165.

44 Jacob H, Kissling R. The mobility of the sacroiliac joints in healthy volunteers between 20 and 50 years of age. Clin Biomechanics 1995;10(7): 352–361.

45 Kissling R, Jacob H. The mobility of the sacroiliac joint in healthy subjects. Bull Hosp Jt Dis 1996; 54(3):158–164.

46 Lund P, Krupinski E, Brooks W. Ultrasound evaluation of sacroiliac motion in normal volunteers. Acad Radiol 1996;3(3):192–196.

47 Wang M, Dumas G. Mechanical behavior of the female sacroiliac joint and influence of the anterior and posterior sacroiliac ligaments under sagittal loads. Clin Biomechanics 1998;13(4/5): 293–299.

48 Sturesson B, Uden A, Vleeming A. A radiostereometric analysis of the movements of the sacroiliac joints in the reciprocal straddle position. Spine 2000;25(2):214–217.

49 Beal MC. The sacroiliac problem: review of anatomy, mechanics, and diagnosis. J Am Osteopath Assoc 1982;81:667–679.

50 McGrath MC. Clinical considerations of sacroiliac joint anatomy: a review of function, motion and pain. J Osteopath Med 2004;7(1):16–24.

51 Kaltenborn F. The Spine. Basic Evaluation and Mobilization Techniques, 2nd edn. Oslo, Norway: Olaf Norlis Bokhandel; 1993.

52 DiGiovanna EL, Schiowitz S. An Osteopathic Approach to Diagnosis and Treatment, 2nd edn. Philadelphia, PA: Lippincott Williams & Wilkins; 1997.

53 Mitchell F, Mitchell P. Muscle Energy Manual, Vol 3: Evaluation and treatment of the pelvis and sacrum. East Lansing, MI: MET; 1999.

54 Greenman PE. Principles of Manual Medicine, 3rd edn. Philadelphia: Lippincott Williams & Wilkins; 2003: 364.

55 Heinking K, Kappler R. Pelvis and sacrum. In: Ward R C ed. Foundations for Osteopathic Medicine, 2nd edn. Philadelphia, PA: Lippincott Williams & Wilkins; 2003:762–783.

56 Stoddard A. Manual of Osteopathic Technique, 2nd edn. London: Hutchinson Medical; 1972.

57 Walton WJ. Textbook of Osteopathic Diagnosis and Technique Procedures, 2nd edn. St Louis, MO: Matthews; 1972.

58 Kimberly PE. Outline of Osteopathic Manipulative Procedures, 2nd edn. Kirksville, MO: Kirksville College of Osteopathic Medicine; 1980.

59 Downing HD. Principles and Practice of Osteopathy. London: Tamor Pierston; 1981.

60 Hartman L. Handbook of Osteopathic Technique, 3rd edn. London: Chapman & Hall; 1997.

61 Kappler R, Jones J. Thrust (high-velocity / low-amplitude) techniques. In: Ward R C ed. Foundations for Osteopathic Medicine. Philadelphia, PA: Lippincott Williams & Wilkins; 2003:852–880.

62 Tullberg T, Blomberg S, Branth B, et al. Manipulation does not alter the position of the sacroiliac joint: a Roentgen stereophotogrammetric analysis. Spine 1998; 23(10):1124–1129.

63 Cibulka MT, Delitto A, Koldehoff RM. Changes in innominate tilt after manipulation of the sacroiliac joint in patients with low back pain. Phys Ther 1988;68(9): 1359–1363.

64 Childs J, Piva S, Erhard R. Immediate improvements in side-to-side weight bearing and iliac crest symmetry after manipulation in patients with low back pain. J Manipulative Physiol Ther 2004;27(5):306–313.

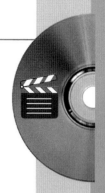

Sacroiliac joint
Left innominate posterior

Patient prone
Ligamentous myofascial tension locking

Assume somatic dysfunction (S-T-A-R-T) is identified and you wish to thrust the left innominate anteriorly.

1. Contact points

(a) Left posterior superior iliac spine (PSIS)
(b) Anterior aspect of left lower thigh.

2. Applicators

(a) Hypothenar eminence of right hand
(b) Palmar aspect of left hand.

3. Patient positioning

Patient lying prone in a comfortable position.

KEY

✳ Stabilization

● Applicator

➜ Plane of thrust (operator)

⇨ Direction of body movement (patient)

Note: The dimensions for the arrows are not a pictorial representation of the amplitude or force of the thrust.

---

4. Operator stance

Stand at the right side of the patient, feet spread slightly and facing the patient. Stand as erect as possible and avoid crouching as this will limit the technique and restrict delivery of the thrust.

5. Palpation of contact points

Place the hypothenar eminence of your right hand against the inferior aspect of the left PSIS. Ensure that you have good contact and will not slip across the skin or superficial musculature. Place the palmar aspect of your left hand gently under the anterior aspect of the left thigh just proximal to the knee.

6. Positioning for thrust

Lift the patient's left leg into extension and slight adduction (Fig. 11.2). Avoid introducing extension into the lumbar spine. Apply a force directed downwards towards the couch and slightly cephalad to fix your right hand against the inferior aspect of the PSIS.

Move your centre of gravity over the patient by leaning your body weight forwards onto your right arm and hypothenar eminence. Shifting your centre of gravity forwards assists firm contact point pressure on the PSIS.

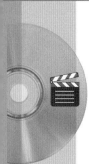

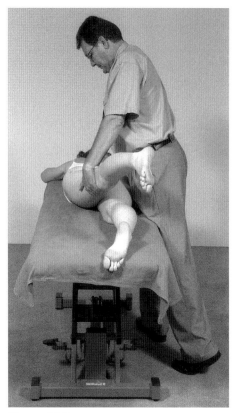

Figure 11.2

7. Adjustments to achieve appropriate pre-thrust tension

Ensure your patient remains relaxed. Maintaining all holds, make any necessary changes in hip extension, adduction and rotation. Simultaneously, adjust the direction of pressure applied to the PSIS until applicator forces are balanced and you sense a state of appropriate tension and leverage at the left sacroiliac joint. The patient should not be aware of any pain or discomfort. Make these final adjustments by slight movements of the shoulders, trunk, ankles, knees and hips.

8. Immediately pre-thrust

Relax and adjust your balance as necessary. Keep your head up and ensure that your contacts are firm. An effective HVLA thrust technique is best achieved if the operator and patient are relaxed and not holding themselves rigid. This is a common impediment to achieving effective cavitation.

9. Delivering the thrust

This technique uses ligamentous myofascial tension locking and not facet apposition locking. This approach generally requires a greater emphasis on the exaggeration of primary leverage than is the case with facet apposition locking techniques.

Apply a HVLA thrust with your right hand directed against the PSIS in a curved plane towards the couch. Simultaneously, apply slight exaggeration of hip extension with your left hand (Fig. 11.3). It is important that you do not overemphasize hip extension at the time of thrust. The aim of this technique is to achieve anterior rotation of the left innominate and movement at the left sacroiliac joint. The direction of thrust will alter from patient to patient as a result of the wide variation in sacroiliac anatomy and biomechanics.

The thrust, although very rapid, must never be excessively forcible. The aim should be to use the absolute minimum force necessary.

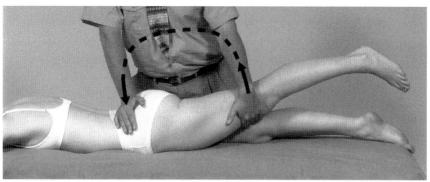
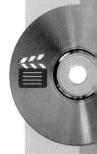

Figure 11.3

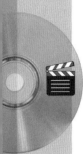

SUMMARY

Sacroiliac joint Left innominate posterior

Patient prone

Thrust anteriorly

Ligamentous myofascial tension locking

- **Contact points:**
  - Left PSIS
  - Anterior aspect of left lower thigh

- **Applicators:**
  - Hypothenar eminence of right hand
  - Palmar aspect of left hand

- **Patient positioning:** Prone in a comfortable position

- **Operator stance:** To right side of patient, facing the couch

- **Palpation of contact points:** Place the hypothenar eminence of your right hand against the inferior aspect of the left PSIS. Place the palmar aspect of your left hand under the anterior aspect of the left thigh proximal to the knee

- **Positioning for thrust:** Lift left leg into extension and slight adduction (Fig. 11.2). Avoid introducing extension into the lumbar spine. Apply a force directed downwards towards the couch and slightly cephalad to fix your right hand against the inferior aspect of the PSIS

- **Adjustments to achieve appropriate pre-thrust tension:** Make any necessary changes in hip extension, adduction and rotation. Simultaneously, adjust the direction of pressure applied to the PSIS

- **Immediately pre-thrust:** Relax and adjust your balance

- **Delivering the thrust:** The thrust against the PSIS is in a curved plane towards the couch and accompanied by slight exaggeration of hip extension (Fig. 11.3)

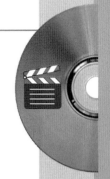

Sacroiliac joint
Right innominate posterior

Patient sidelying

Assume somatic dysfunction (S-T-A-R-T) is identified and you wish to thrust the right innominate anteriorly.

1. **Patient positioning**

Lying on the left side with a pillow to support the head and neck. The upper portion of the couch is raised 30–35° to introduce right sidebending in the lower thoracic and upper lumbar spine.

Lower body. Straighten the patient's lower leg and ensure that the leg and spine are in a straight line, in a neutral position. Flex the patient's upper hip to approximately 90°. Flex the patient's upper knee and place the heel of the foot just anterior to the knee of the lower leg. The lower leg and spine should form as near a straight line as possible with no flexion at the lower hip or knee.

Upper body. Gently extend the patient's upper shoulder and place the patient's right forearm on the lower ribs. Using your left hand to palpate the L5–S1 interspinous space, introduce right rotation of the patient's trunk, down to and including the L5–S1 segment. This is achieved by gently holding the patient's left elbow with your right hand and pulling it towards you, but also in a cephalad direction towards the head end of the couch. Be careful not to introduce any flexion to the spine during this movement. Now modify the pectoral hold by positioning the patient's upper arm behind the thorax.

2. **Operator stance**

Stand close to the couch with your feet spread and one leg behind the other. Ensure that the patient's upper knee is placed between your legs. This will enable you to make the necessary adjustments to achieve the appropriate pre-thrust tension (Fig. 11.4). Maintain an upright posture, facing in the direction of the patient's upper body.

3. **Positioning for thrust**

Apply the heel of your left hand to the inferior aspect of the PSIS. Your right hand should be resting against the patient's upper pectoral and rib cage region. Gently rotate the patient's trunk away from you using your right hand

KEY

❋ Stabilization

● Applicator

→ Plane of thrust (operator)

⇨ Direction of body movement (patient)

Note: The dimensions for the arrows are not a pictorial representation of the amplitude or force of the thrust.

259

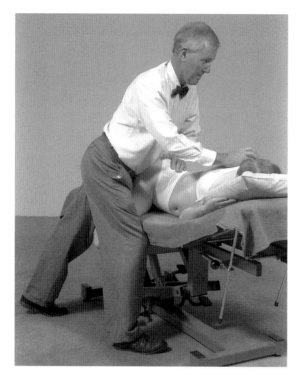

Figure 11.4

until you achieve spinal locking. Avoid applying direct pressure to the glenohumeral joint. Finally, roll the patient about 10–15° towards you while maintaining the build-up of leverages.

4. **Adjustments to achieve appropriate pre-thrust tension**

Ensure your patient remains relaxed. Maintaining all holds, make any necessary changes in hip flexion and adduction. Simultaneously, adjust the direction of pressure applied to the PSIS until the forces are balanced and you sense a state of appropriate tension and leverage at the right sacroiliac joint. The patient should not be aware of any pain or discomfort. Make these final adjustments by slight movements of the shoulders, trunk, ankles, knees and hips.

5. **Immediately pre-thrust**

Relax and adjust your balance as necessary. Keep your head up and ensure your contacts

are firm. An effective HVLA thrust technique is best achieved if the operator and patient are relaxed and not holding themselves rigid. This is a common impediment to achieving effective cavitation.

6. **Delivering the thrust**

Apply a HVLA thrust with the heel of your left hand directed against the PSIS in a curved plane towards you (Fig. 11.5). Your right arm against the patient's pectoral region does not apply a thrust but acts as a stabilizer only. The aim of this technique is to achieve anterior rotation of the right innominate and movement at the right sacroiliac joint. The direction of thrust will alter between patients as a result of the wide variation in sacroiliac anatomy and biomechanics.

The thrust, although very rapid, must never be excessively forcible. The aim should be to use the absolute minimum force necessary.

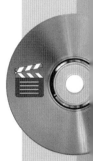

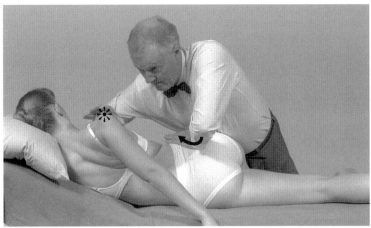

Figure 11.5

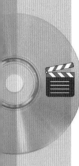

SUMMARY

Sacroiliac joint Right innominate posterior

Patient sidelying

Thrust anteriorly

- **Patient positioning:** Left sidelying with the upper portion of the couch raised 30–35° to introduce right sidebending in the lower thoracic and upper lumbar spine:

  Lower body. Left leg and spine in a straight line. Right hip flexed to approximately 90°. Right knee flexed and heel of right foot placed just anterior to knee of lower leg

  Upper body. Introduce right rotation of the patient's upper body down to and including L5–S1. Do not introduce any flexion to the spine during this movement. Modify the pectoral hold by positioning the patient's upper arm behind the thorax

- **Operator stance:** Stand close to the couch, feet spread and one leg behind the other. Ensure that the patient's upper knee is placed between your legs (Fig. 11.4). Maintain an upright posture facing in the direction of the patient's upper body

- **Positioning for thrust:** Apply the heel of your left hand to the inferior aspect of the PSIS. Rotate the patient's upper body away from you until spinal locking is achieved. Roll the patient about 10–15° towards you

- **Adjustments to achieve appropriate pre-thrust tension:** Make any necessary changes in hip flexion and adduction. Simultaneously, adjust direction of pressure applied to the PSIS

- **Immediately pre-thrust:** Relax and adjust your balance

- **Delivering the thrust:** The thrust against the PSIS is in a curved plane towards you (Fig. 11.5). Your right arm against the patient's pectoral region does not apply a thrust but acts as a stabilizer only

11.3

Sacroiliac joint
Left innominate anterior

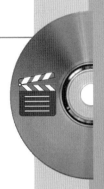

Patient supine

Assume somatic dysfunction (S-T-A-R-T) is identified and you wish to thrust the left innominate posteriorly.

1. **Contact points**

(a) Left anterior superior iliac spine (ASIS)
(b) Posterior aspect of left shoulder girdle.

2. **Applicators**

(a) Palm of right hand
(b) Palmar aspect of left hand and wrist.

3. **Patient positioning**

Patient lying supine in a comfortable position. Move the patient's pelvis towards their right. Move the feet and shoulders in the opposite direction to introduce left sidebending of the trunk. Place the patient's left foot and ankle on top of the right ankle. Ask the patient to clasp their fingers behind the neck (Fig. 11.6).

4. **Operator stance**

Stand at the right side of the patient, feet spread slightly and facing the couch. Stand as erect as possible and avoid crouching as this will limit the technique and restrict delivery of the thrust.

5. **Palpation of contact points**

Place the palm of your right hand over the ASIS. Ensure that you have good contact and will not slip across the skin or superficial musculature. Place the palmar aspect of your left hand and wrist gently over the posterior aspect of the left shoulder girdle.

6. **Positioning for thrust**

Rotate the patient's trunk to the right and towards you. It is critical to maintain the left trunk sidebending introduced during initial positioning. Apply a force directed downwards towards the couch and slightly cephalad to fix your right hand against the inferior aspect of the ASIS (Fig. 11.7).
Move your centre of gravity over the patient by leaning your body weight forwards onto

---

KEY

✳ Stabilization

● Applicator

➜ Plane of thrust (operator)

⇨ Direction of body movement (patient)

Note: The dimensions for the arrows are not a pictorial representation of the amplitude or force of the thrust.

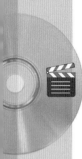

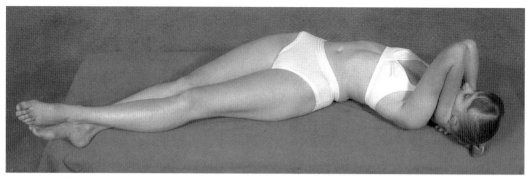

Figure 11.6

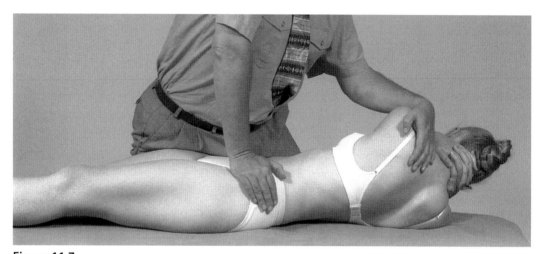

Figure 11.7

your right arm and hand. Shifting your centre of gravity forwards assists firm contact point pressure on the ASIS.

7. **Adjustments to achieve appropriate pre-thrust tension**

Ensure your patient remains relaxed. Maintaining all holds, make any necessary changes in trunk rotation, flexion and sidebending. Simultaneously, adjust the direction of pressure applied to the ASIS until applicator forces are balanced and you sense a state of appropriate tension and leverage. The patient should not be aware of any pain or discomfort. Make these final adjustments by slight movements of the shoulders, trunk, ankles, knees and hips.

8. **Immediately pre-thrust**

Relax and adjust your balance as necessary. Keep your head up and ensure that your contacts are firm. An effective HVLA thrust technique is best achieved if the operator and patient are relaxed and not holding themselves rigid. This is a common impediment to achieving effective cavitation.

9. **Delivering the thrust**

Apply a HVLA thrust with your right hand directed against the ASIS in a curved plane towards the couch (Fig. 11.8). Your left forearm, wrist and hand over the patient's shoulder girdle do not apply a thrust but act as stabilizers only. The aim of this technique is to achieve posterior rotation of the left innominate and movement at the left sacroiliac joint. The direction of thrust will alter between patients as a result of the wide variation in sacroiliac anatomy and biomechanics.

The thrust, although very rapid, must never be excessively forcible. The aim should be to use the absolute minimum force necessary.

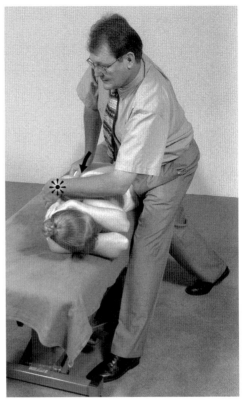
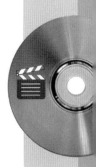

Figure 11.8

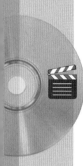

SUMMARY

Sacroiliac joint Left innominate anterior

Patient supine

Thrust posteriorly

- **Contact points:**
  — Left ASIS
  — Posterior aspect of left shoulder girdle

- **Applicators:**
  — Palm of right hand
  — Palmar aspect of left hand and wrist

- **Patient positioning:** Supine. Move patient's pelvis towards the right. Move feet and shoulders in the opposite direction to introduce left sidebending of the trunk. Place the patient's left foot and ankle on top of the right ankle. Ask the patient to clasp fingers behind the neck (Fig. 11.6)

- **Operator stance:** To the right side of the patient, facing the couch

- **Palpation of contact points:** Place the palm of your right hand over the ASIS. Place the palmar aspect of your left hand and wrist over the posterior aspect of the left shoulder girdle

- **Positioning for thrust:** Rotate the patient's trunk to the right. Maintain left trunk sidebending. Apply a force directed downwards towards the couch and slightly cephalad to fix your right hand against the inferior aspect of the ASIS (Fig. 11.7)

- **Adjustments to achieve appropriate pre-thrust tension:** Make any necessary changes in trunk rotation, flexion and sidebending. Simultaneously, adjust direction of pressure applied to the ASIS

- **Immediately pre-thrust:** Relax and adjust your balance

- **Delivering the thrust:** The thrust against the ASIS is in a curved plane towards the couch (Fig. 11.8). Your left forearm, wrist and hand over the patient's shoulder girdle do not apply a thrust but act as stabilizers only

11.4

Sacroiliac joint
Sacral base anterior

Patient sidelying

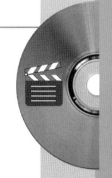

Assume somatic dysfunction (S-T-A-R-T) is identified and you wish to thrust the apex of the sacrum anteriorly.

1. **Patient positioning**

Lying on the right side with a pillow to support the head and neck.

Lower body. Straighten the patient's lower leg and ensure that the leg and spine are in a straight line, in a neutral position. Flex the patient's upper hip and knee slightly and place the upper leg just anterior to the lower leg. The lower leg and spine should form as near a straight line as possible with no flexion at the lower hip or knee.

KEY

✳ Stabilization

● Applicator

→ Plane of thrust (operator)

⇨ Direction of body movement (patient)

Note: The dimensions for the arrows are not a pictorial representation of the amplitude or force of the thrust.

Upper body. Gently extend the patient's upper shoulder and place the patient's left forearm on the lower ribs. Using your right hand to palpate the L5–S1 interspinous space, introduce left rotation of the patient's trunk down to and including the L5–S1 segment. This is achieved by gently holding the patient's right elbow with your left hand and pulling it towards you, but also in a cephalad direction towards the head end of the couch. Be careful not to introduce any flexion to the spine during this movement. Take up the axillary hold. This arm controls and maintains trunk rotation.

2. **Operator stance**

Stand close to the couch with your feet spread and one leg behind the other. Maintain an upright posture, facing slightly in the direction of the patient's upper body.

3. **Positioning for thrust**

Apply the palmar aspect of your right forearm to the apex of the sacrum. Ensure that contact is below the second sacral segment. Your left forearm should be resting against the patient's upper pectoral and rib cage region and will control and maintain trunk rotation. Gently rotate the patient's trunk away from you using your left forearm until you achieve spinal locking. Be careful to avoid undue pressure in the axilla.

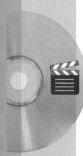

Finally, roll the patient about 10–15° towards you while maintaining the build-up of leverages.

4. **Adjustments to achieve appropriate pre-thrust tension**

Ensure your patient remains relaxed. Maintaining all holds, make any necessary changes in flexion, extension, sidebending or rotation until you are confident that full spinal locking is achieved. The patient should not be aware of any pain or discomfort. Make these final adjustments by slight movements of your shoulders, trunk, ankles, knees and hips.

5. **Immediately pre-thrust**

Relax and adjust your balance as necessary. Keep your head up and ensure contacts are firm. An effective HVLA thrust technique is best achieved if both the operator and patient are relaxed and not holding themselves rigid. This is a common impediment to achieving effective cavitation.

6. **Delivering the thrust**

Apply a HVLA thrust with your right forearm against the apex of the sacrum in a curved plane towards you (Fig. 11.9). Your left arm against the patient's pectoral region does not apply a thrust but acts as a stabilizer only. The aim of this technique is to achieve a counter-nutation movement of the sacrum.

The thrust, although very rapid, must never be excessively forcible. The aim should be to use the absolute minimum force necessary.

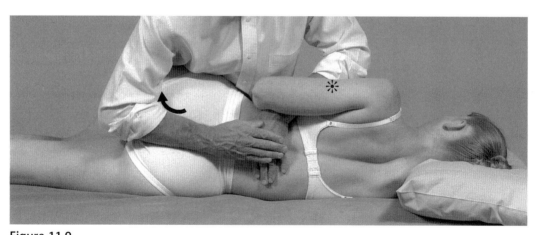

Figure 11.9

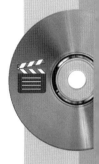

SUMMARY

Sacroiliac joint Sacral base anterior

Patient sidelying

Thrust apex anteriorly

- **Patient positioning:** Right sidelying:

    Lower body. Right leg and spine in a straight line. Left hip and knee flexed slightly and placed just anterior to the lower leg

    Upper body. Introduce left rotation of the patient's trunk down to and including the L5–S1 segment. Do not introduce any flexion to the spine during this movement. Take up the axillary hold

- **Operator stance:** Stand close to the couch, feet spread and one leg behind the other. Maintain an upright posture, facing slightly in the direction of the patient's upper body

- **Positioning for thrust:** Apply the palmar aspect of your right forearm to the apex of the sacrum. Ensure that contact is below the second sacral segment. Your left forearm should be resting against the patient's upper pectoral and rib cage region. Rotate the patient's trunk away from you using your left forearm until you achieve spinal locking. Roll the patient about 10–15° towards you

- **Adjustments to achieve appropriate pre-thrust tension**

- **Immediately pre-thrust:** Relax and adjust your balance

- **Delivering the thrust:** The thrust against the apex of the sacrum is in a curved plane towards you (Fig. 11.9). Your left arm against the patient's pectoral region does not apply a thrust but acts as a stabilizer only

Sacrococcygeal joint
Coccyx anterior

Patient sidelying

Assume somatic dysfunction (S-T-A-R-T) is identified and you wish to thrust the coccyx posteriorly.

The operator must exercise care and attention to ensure that the patient is fully informed as to the nature of this procedure. This technique involves both assessment and treatment via a rectal approach. It is assumed that the operator will examine the anal and rectal region to determine if there are any contraindications to performing this procedure. This technique can be used either as a means of gently articulating the sacrococcygeal joint or applying a HVLA thrust to the coccyx. Coccydynia can be severe and the choice of technique depends as much upon patient comfort as perceived efficacy of approach. Practitioners should become familiar with articulating the sacrococcygeal joint before attempting a thrust to the coccyx.

1. Contact points

(a) Anterior aspect of the coccyx through the posterior wall of the rectum
(b) Posterior aspect of the coccyx.

2. Applicators

(a) Lubricated index finger of operator's gloved right hand
(b) Thumb of operator's gloved right hand.

3. Patient positioning

Lying in the left lateral position with the maximal amount of flexion of the hips, knees and spine consistent with patient comfort. The patient should be fully undressed so that access to the anal canal is possible. The buttocks should be at the edge of the couch.

4. Operator stance

Stand behind the patient, approximately at the level of the patient's hip joints, facing the couch and patient's back.

5. Palpation of contact points

The operator should be wearing a pair of suitable gloves with lubricant smeared over

---

KEY

❊ Stabilization

● Applicator

➜ Plane of thrust (operator)

⇨ Direction of body movement (patient)

Note: The dimensions for the arrows are not a pictorial representation of the amplitude or force of the thrust.

the right index finger. The patient must be informed that a finger within the rectum will cause a sensation similar to that of opening the bowels. Ask the patient to relax and place the index finger of your right hand against the anal margin (Fig. 11.10A). With steady pressure, insert your right index finger into the patient's anal canal in a cephalic and slightly anterior direction (Fig. 11.10B). The finger will pass through the anal sphincter and into the rectum. If the patient has difficulty relaxing, ask him / her to bear down as if opening the bowels and gently slip your finger past the anal sphincter and into the rectum. Once through the anal sphincter, the direction of the rectum is cephalic and posteriorly along the curve of the coccyx and sacrum. At this stage an examination of the rectum should be undertaken. For male patients this would include examination of the prostate gland.

The palpating right index finger identifies the sacrum and coccyx through the posterior wall of the rectum. Place the distal phalanx of the right index finger against the anterior surface of the coccyx immediately below the sacrococcygeal joint. Use the thumb of your right hand externally to identify the posterior aspect of the coccyx between the buttocks. The coccyx is now gently held between your index finger internally and thumb externally (Fig. 11.10C). Gentle pressure is applied in a number of directions to determine undue tenderness or any reproduction of the patient's familiar symptoms. The mobility and position of the coccyx relative to the sacrum is also noted.

6. Fixation of contact points

Keep your right index finger on the anterior aspect of the coccyx while applying pressure against the posterior aspect of the coccyx with your right thumb. The fixation is gentle but firm with less pressure against the anterior surface of the coccyx.

7. Adjustments to achieve appropriate pre-thrust tension

The operator should be in a position to move the coccyx through a range of motion and in different planes. Ensure your patient remains relaxed. Maintaining all holds, make any necessary changes in flexion, extension,

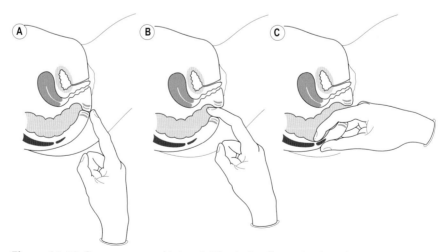

Figure 11.10 Sacrococcygeal joint. A: The index finger is placed against the anal margin. B: The finger is inserted as shown. C: After examination of the rectum, the coccyx is held between the index finger internally and the thumb externally.

sidebending and rotation of the coccyx until you sense a state of appropriate tension and leverage at the sacrococcygeal joint.

8. **Immediately pre-thrust**

Relax and adjust your balance as necessary. Ensure that your contacts are firm. An effective HVLA thrust technique is best achieved if the operator and patient are relaxed and not holding themselves rigid. This is a common impediment to achieving effective cavitation.

9. **Delivering the thrust**

Apply a HVLA thrust towards you in a curved plane (Fig. 11.11).

The thrust, although very rapid, must never be excessively forcible. The aim should be to use the absolute minimum force necessary.

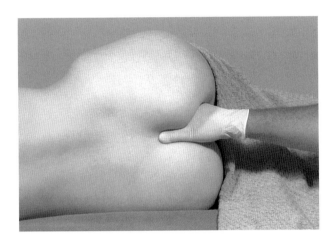

Figure 11.11

SUMMARY

Sacrococcygeal joint Coccyx anterior

Patient sidelying

Thrust posteriorly

- **Contact points:**
  - — Anterior aspect of the coccyx
  - — Posterior aspect of the coccyx

- **Applicators:**
  - — Lubricated index finger of operator's gloved right hand
  - — Thumb of operator's gloved right hand

- **Patient positioning:** Left lateral position with flexion of the hips, knees and spine

- **Operator stance:** Behind the patient

- **Palpation of contact points:** Place the index finger of right hand against the anal margin (Fig. 11.10A). Insert your right index finger into the anal canal in a cephalic and anterior direction (Fig. 11.10B). The palpating index finger identifies the sacrum and coccyx through the posterior wall of the rectum. Place the distal phalanx of the right index finger against the anterior surface of the coccyx. Identify the posterior aspect of the coccyx between the buttocks. The coccyx is now gently held between your right index finger internally and thumb externally (Fig. 11.10C)

- **Fixation of contact points:** Keep right index finger on the anterior aspect of the coccyx while applying pressure against the posterior aspect of the coccyx with your right thumb

- **Adjustments to achieve appropriate pre-thrust tension**

- **Immediately pre-thrust:** Relax and adjust your balance

- **Delivering the thrust:** The direction of thrust is towards you in a curved plane (Fig. 11.11)

Technique failure and analysis

Techniques in this manual have been described in a structured format. This format allows flexibility so that each technique can be modified to suit both the patient and practitioner.

Competence and expertise in the use of high-velocity low-amplitude (HVLA) thrust techniques increase with practice and experience. Development of a high level of skill in the use of HVLA thrust techniques is predicated upon critical reflection of performance. When a HVLA thrust technique does not produce cavitation with minimal force, the practitioner should reflect upon how the technique might have been modified and improved. Even the experienced practitioner should review each HVLA thrust technique to identify factors that might improve technique delivery.

Inability to achieve cavitation with minimal force may arise for a number of reasons and can be reviewed under three broad headings:

- *General technique analysis*
  - Incorrect selection of technique
  - Inadequate localization of forces
  - Ineffective thrust
- *Practitioner and patient variables*
  - Patient comfort and cooperation
  - Patient positioning
  - Practitioner comfort and confidence
  - Practitioner posture
- *Physical and biomechanical modifying factors*
  - Primary leverage
  - Secondary leverages
  - Contact point pressure
  - Identification of appropriate pre-thrust tension
  - Direction of thrust
  - Velocity of thrust
  - Amplitude of thrust
  - Force of thrust
  - Arrest of technique.

If you have experienced technique failure, follow the process of review outlined below:

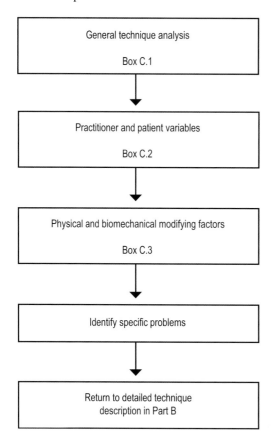

```
┌─────────────────────────────────┐
│   General technique analysis    │
│                                 │
│           Box C.1               │
└─────────────────────────────────┘
                 │
                 ▼
┌─────────────────────────────────┐
│ Practitioner and patient variables │
│                                 │
│           Box C.2               │
└─────────────────────────────────┘
                 │
                 ▼
┌─────────────────────────────────┐
│ Physical and biomechanical modifying factors │
│                                 │
│           Box C.3               │
└─────────────────────────────────┘
                 │
                 ▼
┌─────────────────────────────────┐
│    Identify specific problems   │
└─────────────────────────────────┘
                 │
                 ▼
┌─────────────────────────────────┐
│  Return to detailed technique   │
│    description in Part B        │
└─────────────────────────────────┘
```

Box C.1 General technique analysis

Incorrect selection of technique
- Practitioner too small and patient too large
- Practitioner has physical limitations that limit effective delivery of technique
- Practitioner inexperienced with selected technique
- Inability to position patient due to pain, discomfort or physical limitations
- Patient apprehension

Inadequate localization of forces
- Incorrect application of primary leverage
- Incorrect application of secondary leverages
- Inability to recognize appropriate pre-thrust tension

Ineffective thrust
- Loss of contact point pressure
- Poor bimanual coordination
- Incorrect direction of thrust
- Inadequate velocity of thrust
- Incorrect amplitude of thrust
- Incorrect force of thrust
- Loss of leverage at time of thrust
- Poor practitioner posture
- Practitioner not relaxed
- Failure to arrest thrust and leverage adequately
- Lack of practitioner confidence

Box C.2 Practitioner and patient variables

Common faults
- Patient not comfortably positioned
- Patient not relaxed
- Rough patient handling
- Rushing technique
- Poor practitioner posture
- Lack of practitioner confidence

Checklist
Patient comfort and cooperation
Dependent upon:
- Confidence and trust in practitioner
- Patient experience of previous successful HVLA thrust technique
- Slow, firm and gentle patient handling
- Confident and reassuring approach by practitioner
- Explanation of technique and informed consent
- Optimal patient positioning

Patient positioning
Dependent upon:
- Appropriate positioning to match patient's physical and medical condition
- Correct identification of primary leverage and secondary leverages
- Pain-free positioning
- Appropriate use of pillows and treatment couch adjustment

Practitioner comfort and confidence
Dependent upon:
- Establishing a working diagnosis
- Selecting a technique to match patient's physical and medical condition
- Confidence that the technique will improve and not worsen the patient's symptoms
- Previous experience and success with the selected HVLA thrust technique
- Optimal practitioner posture

Practitioner posture
Dependent upon:
- Using as wide a base as possible
- Not relying solely upon arm strength and speed
- Using your body where possible to generate thrust force
- Not stooping or bending over the patient
- Keeping your own spine erect
- Optimal treatment couch height

Box C.3 Physical and biomechanical modifying factors

Common faults
- Insufficient primary leverage
- Too much secondary leverage – locking often results from the over-application of secondary leverages. This can occur during the build-up of leverages or at the point of thrust
- Loss of contact point pressure immediately pre-thrust
- Not identifying appropriate pre-thrust tension and leverage prior to thrust – if in doubt about optimum pre-thrust tension, attempt multiple light thrusts
- Incorrect direction of thrust – the thrust should be in a direction that is comfortable for the patient. Multiple light thrusts can assist in the identification of the appropriate direction of thrust
- Insufficient velocity of thrust
- Too much amplitude – this is often a consequence of too much force and/or poor control
- Too much force
- Insufficient arrest of technique – this is often a consequence of poor practitioner coordination and control

Checklist
- Primary leverage
- Secondary leverages
- Contact point pressure
- Identification of appropriate pre-thrust tension
- Direction of thrust
- Velocity of thrust
- Amplitude of thrust
- Force of thrust
- Arrest of technique

Index

ELSEVIER DVD-ROM LICENCE AGREEMENT

and of the Proprietary Material, together with any and all accompanying documentation. All provisions relating to proprietary rights shall survive termination of this Agreement.

LIMITED WARRANTY AND LIMITATION OF LIABILITY

Elsevier warrants that the software embodied in this Product will perform in substantial compliance with the documentation supplied in this Product, unless the performance problems are the result of hardware failure or improper use. If You report a significant defect in performance in writing to Elsevier within ninety (90) calendar days of your having purchased the Product, and Elsevier is not able to correct same within sixty (60) days after its receipt of Your notification, You may return this Product, including all copies and documentation, to Elsevier and Elsevier will refund Your money. In order to apply for a refund on your purchased Product, please contact the return address on the invoice to obtain the refund request form ('Refund Request Form'), and either fax or mail your signed request and your proof of purchase to the address indicated on the Refund Request Form. Incomplete forms will not be processed. Defined terms in the Refund Request Form shall have the same meaning as in this Agreement.

YOU UNDERSTAND THAT, EXCEPT FOR THE LIMITED WARRANTY RECITED ABOVE, ELSEVIER, ITS AFFILIATES, LICENSORS, THIRD PARTY SUPPLIERS AND AGENTS (TOGETHER 'THE SUPPLIERS') MAKE NO REPRESENTATIONS OR WARRANTIES, WITH RESPECT TO THE PRODUCT, INCLUDING, WITHOUT LIMITATION THE PROPRIETARY MATERIAL. ALL OTHER REPRESENTATIONS, WARRANTIES, CONDITIONS OR OTHER TERMS, WHETHER EXPRESS OR IMPLIED BY STATUTE OR COMMON LAW, ARE HEREBY EXCLUDED TO THE FULLEST EXTENT PERMITTED BY LAW.

IN PARTICULAR BUT WITHOUT LIMITATION TO THE FOREGOING NONE OF THE SUPPLIERS MAKE ANY REPRESENTIONS OR WARRANTIES (WHETHER EXPRESS OR IMPLIED) REGARDING THE PERFORMANCE OF YOUR PAD, NETWORK OR COMPUTER SYSTEM WHEN USED IN CONJUNCTION WITH THE PRODUCT, NOR THAT THE PRODUCT WILL MEET YOUR REQUIREMENTS OR THAT ITS OPERATION WILL BE UNINTERRUPTED OR ERROR-FREE.

EXCEPT IN RESPECT OF DEATH OR PERSONAL INJURY CAUSED BY THE SUPPLIERS' NEGLIGENCE AND TO THE FULLEST EXTENT PERMITTED BY LAW, IN NO EVENT (AND REGARDLESS OF WHETHER SUCH DAMAGES ARE FORESEEABLE AND OF WHETHER SUCH LIABILITY IS BASED IN TORT, CONTRACT OR OTHERWISE) WILL ANY OF THE SUPPLIERS BE LIABLE TO YOU FOR ANY DAMAGES (INCLUDING, WITHOUT LIMITATION, ANY LOST PROFITS, LOST SAVINGS OR OTHER SPECIAL, INDIRECT, INCIDENTAL OR CONSEQUENTIAL DAMAGES ARISING OUT OF OR RESULTING FROM: (I) YOUR USE OF, OR INABILITY TO USE, THE PRODUCT; (II) DATA LOSS OR CORRUPTION; AND/OR (III) ERRORS OR OMISSIONS IN THE PROPRIETARY MATERIAL.

IF THE FOREGOING LIMITATION IS HELD TO BE UNENFORCEABLE, OUR MAXIMUM LIABILITY TO YOU IN RESPECT THEREOF SHALL NOT EXCEED THE AMOUNT OF THE LICENCE FEE PAID BY YOU FOR THE PRODUCT. THE REMEDIES AVAILABLE TO YOU AGAINST ELSEVIER AND THE LICENSORS OF MATERIALS INCLUDED IN THE PRODUCT ARE EXCLUSIVE.

If the information provided in the Product contains medical or health sciences information, it is intended for professional use within the medical field. Information about medical treatment or drug dosages is intended strictly for professional use, and because of rapid advances in the medical sciences, independent verification of diagnosis and drug dosages should be made.

The provisions of this Agreement shall be severable, and in the event that any provision of this Agreement is found to be legally unenforceable, such unenforceability shall not prevent the enforcement or any other provision of this Agreement.

GOVERNING LAW

This Agreement shall be governed by the laws of England and Wales. In any dispute arising out of this Agreement, you and Elsevier each consent to the exclusive personal jurisdiction and venue in the courts of England and Wales.